Arterial Blood Gas interpretation:
A case study approach

Full the full range of M&K Publishing books please visit our website:
www.mkupdate.co.uk

Arterial Blood Gas interpretation
A case study approach

Edited by Mark Ranson and Donna Pierre

Arterial Blood Gas interpretation: A case study approach

Mark Ranson

Donna Pierre

ISBN: 978-1-905539-98-7

First published 2016

British Library Catalogue in Publication Data
A catalogue record for this book is available from the British Library

Notice
Clinical practice and medical knowledge constantly evolve. Standard safety precautions must be followed, but, as knowledge is broadened by research, changes in practice, treatment and drug therapy may become necessary or appropriate. Readers must check the most current product information provided by the manufacturer of each drug to be administered and verify the dosages and correct administration, as well as contraindications. It is the responsibility of the practitioner, utilising the experience and knowledge of the patient, to determine dosages and the best treatment for each individual patient. Any brands mentioned in this book are as examples only and are not endorsed by the Publisher. Neither the publisher nor the authors assume any liability for any injury and/or damage to persons or property arising from this publication.

Disclaimer
M&K Publishing cannot accept responsibility for the contents of any linked website or online resource. The existence of a link does not imply any endorsement or recommendation of the organisation or the information or views which may be expressed in any linked website or online resource. We cannot guarantee that these links will operate consistently and we have no control over the availability of linked pages.

The Publisher
To contact M&K Publishing write to:
M&K Update Ltd · The Old Bakery · St. John's Street
Keswick · Cumbria CA12 5AS
Tel: 01768 773030 · Fax: 01768 781099
publishing@mkupdate.co.uk
www.mkupdate.co.uk

Designed and typeset by Mary Blood
Printed in Scotland by Bell & Bain, Glasgow

Contents

About the contributors

Dawn Parsons MA, PGCE, BSc (Hons), DipHE, RGN, EN

Dawn became a registered general nurse in Suffolk in 1995 and worked as a staff nurse in various ward areas, including gynaecology, acute medicine and oncology. Since 2010, she has been a lecturer in the Acute and Critical Care team at University Campus Suffolk. During this time, she has developed her skills in teaching, learning and assessing for operating department practitioners and both pre- and post-registration nurses. For the last few years, she has been the deputy course leader for the DipHE in Operating Department Practice.

Donna Pierre PGCHE, MSc Advanced Nurse Practitioner, RGN

After qualifying as a registered adult nurse in 2003, Donna started her career on a surgical vascular ward, at a major trauma centre in London. After three years, she developed an interest in critical care nursing, in which she still works – in areas such as trauma, cardiac care, haematology and oncology, neurovascular and head injury, liver, and paediatric critical care. She joined the University of Suffolk in 2012, and contributes to pre-registration and post-registration nursing programmes, operating department practitioner programmes and paramedic programmes. She now leads the BSc in Adult Nursing (Work-based Learning Pathway) and the BA in Health and Social Care.

Mark Ranson MA, PGCE, BSc (Hons), Specialist Practitioner (NMC), Dip HE, RGN

As a registered nurse with over 20 years' experience in healthcare, Mark has worked in a variety of clinical settings, including acute respiratory medicine, critical care and cardiology. Following a successful clinical career, Mark moved into a lecturing role and now leads and contributes to a wide range of healthcare educational programmes, including pre-registration nursing, post-registration nursing, operating department practice and paramedic science. Mark's particular field of academic interest is Advanced Healthcare Practice. He is a senior lecturer in Acute and Critical Care at University Campus Suffolk.

Stanley Swanepoel PGCE HE, BSc (Hons), RODP

After completing professional training in Peterborough (Cambridgeshire), in 1987, based at the Peterborough District Hospital, Stanley worked at De La Pole Hospital at an elective orthopaedic unit for six months. This was followed by a move to Norwich, where the next 25 years were spent predominantly in the orthopaedic and trauma theatres. The enjoyment of teaching students in practice eventually led him to move into full-time teaching and he now leads the Operating Department Practice course at the University of Suffolk.

1

Introduction to acid-base balance

Mark Ranson

The homeostatic control of hydrogen ion concentration in body fluids is an essential requirement for life – to defend the relatively alkaline environment required for the most efficient maintenance of body processes and organ function (Ayers & Dixon 2012). The degree of acidity or alkalinity of a solution is dictated by the pH (potential of hydrogen ion concentration). Large quantities of volatile acids are produced from cellular metabolism (mainly carbon dioxide – CO_2), and non-volatile acids from the metabolism of fats and certain proteins. A robust system for the maintenance of plasma pH is therefore required to defend the alkaline environment in the face of this massive, daily acid load.

An acid, by definition, is a substance that can donate (give up) hydrogen (H^+) ions. A strong acid donates a lot of hydrogen ions, while a weak acid will donate only a few. An alkaline (or base) is a substance that can accept (take up) H^+ ions. Like an acid, a strong alkali can accept a lot of H^+ ions, while a weak one can only accept a few. The pH is related to the actual H^+ concentration. A low pH corresponds to a high H^+ concentration and is evidence of an acidosis. Conversely, a high pH corresponds to a low H^+ concentration, known as an alkalosis (Edwards 2008). The interrelationship between oxygen (O_2), H^+, CO_2 and bicarbonate (HCO_3^-) is central to the understanding of acid-base balance. It also reflects the physiological importance of the CO_2/HCO_3^- buffer system, as illustrated in Figure 1.1 (below).

$$CO_2 + H_2O \leftrightarrow H_2CO_3 \leftrightarrow H^+ + HCO_3^-$$

CO_2 = carbon dioxide; H_2O = water; H_2CO_3 = carbonic acid; H^+ = hydrogen; HCO_3^- = bicarbonate

Figure 1.1 The interrelationship between H^+, CO_2 and HCO_3^- in acid-base balance

Mechanisms that maintain normal pH values

Maintenance of plasma pH within the range 7.35–7.45 is an essential requirement for life because many metabolic processes (such as enzymatic reactions) are extremely sensitive to changes in H^+

concentration. Intracellular H^+ concentration is higher (around pH 7.00) than that in extracellular fluid (ECF), but is sensitive to changes in extracellular H^+ concentration. In terms of total volatile acid production, CO_2 provides the largest contribution at 15–20mmol/day. This can occur either by the hydration of CO_2 to form the weak, volatile carbonic acid or by hydroxylation of CO_2 following the splitting of water. The products of both of these reactions are H^+ and HCO_3^-.

Non-volatile acids contribute much less to daily acid production. Such acids include sulphuric acid from sulphur-containing amino acids, hydrochloric acid from cationic amino acids and phosphoric acid from the metabolism of phospholipids and phosphorylated amino acids. The contribution of non-volatile acids to daily acid production depends on dietary intake. If meat is a major component of the diet, non-volatile acids are significant (about 50mmol/day), whereas this is much lower if the diet is mainly composed of fruit and vegetables (Rogers & McCutcheon 2013).

Three basic mechanisms exist in order to defend and maintain the pH within functional parameters:

- Physicochemical buffering
- Respiratory compensation
- Renal compensation.

Physicochemical buffering takes place via the main buffer systems in body fluids. These include: plasma proteins, haemoglobin and bicarbonate in the blood; bicarbonate in the interstitial fluid; and proteins and phosphates in the intracellular fluid. These buffering mechanisms are instantaneous but only limit the fall in pH.

Respiratory compensation is rapid (taking place in minutes) and operates via the control of plasma partial pressure of CO_2 (pCO_2) through changes in alveolar ventilation and subsequent excretion of CO_2. Although this will allow the plasma pH to be returned towards normal values, this system cannot completely correct the acid-base balance.

Renal compensation is slower (taking place over hours or days) and operates via the control of plasma bicarbonate through changes in the renal secretion of H^+, reabsorption and production of bicarbonate. This final mechanism facilitates complete correction of acid-base balance.

Normal blood gas values

Normal blood gas values for arterial and venous blood are shown in Table 1.1 (below). Arterial blood gas measurement provides an indication of the lungs' ability to oxygenate the blood whilst venous blood gas measurement can give an indication of the efficiency of tissue oxygenation.

Table 1.1 Reference blood gas values

	Arterial blood	Venous blood
pH	7.35–7.45	7.31–7.41
PaCO$_2$ (kPa)	4.6–6.0	5.5–6.8
PaO$_2$ (kPa)	12.0–14.5	4.6–5.8
Bicarbonate – HCO$_3^-$ (MEq/l)	22–26	22–26
Base excess	-2 to +2	-2 to +2
O$_2$ saturation	95% +	70–75%

Key: kPa = kilopascals; MEq/l = milliequivalents per litre

The oxygen dissociation curve

The oxygen dissociation curve is a graph that shows the percentage saturation of haemoglobin (Hb) at various partial pressures of oxygen, as illustrated in Figure 1.2 (below).

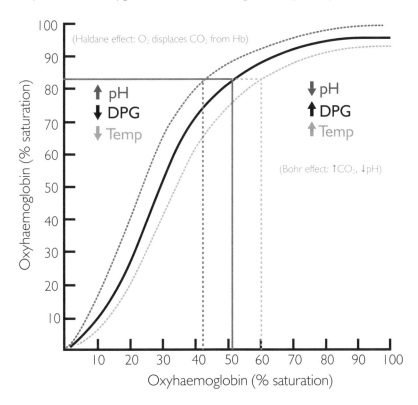

Figure 1.2 Oxyhaemoglobin dissociation curve

The purpose of the oxygen dissociation curve is to show the equilibrium of oxyhaemoglobin and non-bonded haemoglobin at various partial pressures. At high partial pressures of oxygen, haemoglobin binds to oxygen to form oxyhaemoglobin. When the blood is fully saturated, all the red blood cells are in the form of oxyhaemoglobin. As the red blood cells travel to tissues deprived of oxygen, the partial pressure of oxygen will decrease. As a consequence of this, the oxyhaemoglobin releases the oxygen to form haemoglobin.

The shape of the oxygen dissociation curve is a product of binding of the oxygen to the four polypeptide chains. A characteristic of haemoglobin is that it has a greater ability to bind oxygen once a sub-unit has bound oxygen. Haemoglobin is therefore most attracted to oxygen when three of the four polypeptide chains are bound to oxygen. This is known as co-operative binding (Aiken 2013).

The binding of oxygen to haemoglobin can be influenced by a number of factors. An increase in body temperature can denature the bond between oxygen and haemoglobin, thus increasing the amounts of oxygen and haemoglobin but decreasing the amount of bound oxyhaemoglobin. This causes a right shift in the oxygen dissociation curve.

A Bohr shift is characterised by more oxygen being given up as oxygen pressure rises. A decrease in the pH (by the addition of carbon dioxide or other acids) causes a Bohr shift and the oxygen dissociation curve shifts to the right. The main primary organic phosphate in the body is 2, 3-diphosphoglycerate (DPG). DPG can bind to haemoglobin, which decreases the affinity of oxygen for haemoglobin, causing a right shift in the oxygen dissociation curve (Day & Pandit 2010).

Carbon monoxide (CO) combines with haemoglobin to form carboxyhaemoglobin (COHb). CO has a much higher affinity for haemoglobin than O_2, and this means that a small amount of CO can tie up a large percentage of the haemoglobin in the blood, which renders the Hb unavailable to carry oxygen. This can result in a normal presentation of PaO_2 and Hb concentration but with a grossly reduced O_2 concentration. The presence of COHb also causes a left shift in the oxygen dissociation curve, interfering with the unloading of O_2 to the tissues. All these factors contribute to the toxic effects of CO.

How does the blood transport O_2 and CO_2?

The blood's function in transporting O_2 and CO_2 plays a significant role in maintaining blood pH. This is because the rate at which Hb can reversibly bind with, or release, O_2 is regulated by factors such as the PaO_2, the temperature, the blood pH and the PCO_2.

Blood carries O_2 in two main ways. In normal physiology, almost all the oxygen (97%) is bound to haemoglobin, forming oxyhaemoglobin (HbO_2). The remaining 3% is dissolved in the plasma for transport. Each Hb molecule can combine with four molecules of O_2. After the first molecule binds, the haemoglobin molecule changes shape, facilitating the uptake of three further O_2 molecules, until all four are saturated, resulting in full saturation. At the tissues, the unloading of one O_2 molecule enhances the unloading of the next, until all four molecules are released.

Blood carries CO_2 in three main ways, with 60–70% being converted to bicarbonate ions and transported in the plasma. Around 20–30% binds with Hb in the red blood cells, with the remaining small percentage being dissolved in the plasma. CO_2 rapidly dissociates from Hb in the lungs, where the PCO_2 of alveolar air is lower than in the blood. Deoxygenated Hb has a much greater affinity for CO_2 (known as the Haldane effect), thus facilitating removal of CO_2 from the tissues (Atherton 2009).

Changes in respiratory rate or depth can produce dramatic changes in the blood pH. Slow, shallow respiration can result in an increased level of CO_2 in the blood and blood pH therefore drops. Conversely, rapid and deep breathing can result in a decreased level of CO_2 in the blood and the blood pH consequently rises. These changes in respiratory ventilation can thus provide a fast-acting method to adjust blood pH (and PCO_2) when they are disturbed by disease.

The human body contains a number of chemical buffers that resist changes in pH when a strong acid or base is introduced into the system. In general terms, the buffers achieve this by binding to hydrogen ions when the pH drops, and releasing them when the pH rises.

The bicarbonate buffer system (outlined in Figure 1.1, p. 1) plays a primary role in preventing pH changes caused by organic acids and fixed acids in the extracellular fluid. For example, if there is an increase in CO_2, as in chronic obstructive pulmonary disease (COPD), respiratory acid is buffered by bicarbonate, thus reducing the levels of HCO_3^- in the blood.

The phosphate buffer system is similar to the bicarbonate buffer system, with different components – dihydrogen phosphate which acts as a weak acid; and monohydrogen phosphate which acts as a weak base. This buffer system plays only a secondary role in the regulation of pH, as the concentration of bicarbonate far outweighs that of the phosphate system. The phosphate system does, however, play an important role in the buffering of pH in the intracellular fluid (ICF).

Finally, the protein buffer system exists but this is a slow process that depends on the ability of amino acids to respond to alterations in pH by releasing or accepting hydrogen. If the pH of the extracellular fluid (ECF) decreases, the cells pump hydrogen out of the extracellular fluid and into the intracellular fluid, where they can be buffered by intracellular proteins. If the pH of the extracellular fluid rises, exchange pumps located in cell membranes can exchange hydrogen in the intracellular fluids for potassium in the extracellular fluid. This buffer system can help to prevent major changes in the pH when plasma CO_2 level is rising or falling.

The kidneys play a major role in the regulation of acid-base balance by acting slowly to compensate for acid-base imbalances caused by diet, metabolism or disease. The major renal mechanisms for regulating acid-base involve the excretion of bicarbonate ions and the conservation (reabsorption) of hydrogen ions in alkalotic states. Conversely, in acidotic states, the kidneys play an important role by excreting hydrogen ions and reclaiming (reabsorbing) bicarbonate ions (Ayers *et al.* 2015).

Many systemic conditions leading to ill health can result in disturbances in acid-base balance. In altered physiology, a low pH corresponds to a high hydrogen concentration and is known as an acidosis. A high pH corresponds to a low hydrogen concentration and is known as an alkalosis. In essence, if acid production is lower than acid excretion, bicarbonate increases and hydrogen reduces, resulting in an alkalosis with a corresponding increase in pH. If acid production is greater than excretion, then hydrogen increases and bicarbonate decreases, resulting in an acidosis with a corresponding decrease in pH. Acid-base disorders are generally associated with metabolic disorders where there are changes in bicarbonate, or respiratory disorders from an accumulation or reduction of PCO_2 (an acid that increases hydrogen concentrations).

By measuring the partial pressure of gases and other parameters in arterial and/or venous blood, we can determine whether acidosis or alkalosis is present. Arterial blood gas analysis can also help to determine whether the acid-base imbalance is respiratory or metabolic, and establish whether the kidneys are attempting to compensate for the condition. With all this in mind, the healthcare professional's ability to accurately interpret arterial blood gas results is clearly very important in order to respond appropriately, and in a timely manner, to acid-base balance disturbances.

References

Aiken, C.G.A. (2013). History and medical understanding and misunderstanding of acid base balance. *Journal of Clinical and Diagnostic Research.* **7**(9), 2038–41.

Atherton, J.C. (2009 Acid-base balance: maintenance of plasma pH. *Anaesthesia and Intensive Care.* **10**(11), 557–61

Ayers, P. & Dixon, C. (2012). Simple acid-base tutorial. *Journal of Parenteral and Enteral Nutrition.* **36**(1), 18–23.

Ayers, P., Dixon, C. & Mays, A. (2015). Acid-base disorders: Learning the basics. *Nutrition in Clinical Practice.* **30**(1), 14–20.

Day, J. & Pandit, J.J. (2010). Analysis of blood gases and acid-base balance. *Surgery.* **29**(3), 107–11.

Edwards, S.L. (2008). Pathophysiology of acid base balance: The theory practice relationship. *Intensive and Critical Care Nursing.* **24**, 28–40

Rogers, K.M.A. & McCutcheon, K. (2013). Understanding arterial blood gases. *The Journal of Perioperative Practice.* **23**(9), 191–97

2

A systematic approach to ABG interpretation

Donna Pierre

Step 1: Review the patient

In order to interpret an ABG, consideration must be given to the patient's presenting complaint, clinical history and physical examination, as patients may show some signs and symptoms that have developed as a result of the disturbance.

Step 2: Analyse the oxygenation

SaO$_2$

As mentioned earlier, 97% of O$_2$ is transported in the blood, bound to haemoglobin (as oxyhaemoglobin), while the remaining 3% is transported dissolved in blood plasma (Lynch 2009). SaO$_2$, or oxygen saturation, is a direct measurement of the ratio of oxygen bound to haemoglobin (expressed as a percentage) and is the key means of transporting oxygen to the tissue cells. The normal SaO$_2$ range is 92–98%, and should always be compared with FiO$_2$, to ensure that the SaO$_2$ is within normal range.

PaO$_2$

The partial pressure of oxygen (PaO$_2$) is the amount of oxygen dissolved in the blood, and reflects gas exchange in the lungs. The normal PaO$_2$ should be greater than 10.6kPa (79.5mmHg). If it is lower than expected, indicating hypoxemia, it is often as a result of hypoventilation or a ventilation perfusion mismatch (Verma & Roach 2010), indicating a type 1 respiratory failure (PaO$_2$ <8kPa (60mmHg). If hypoxemia is associated with an increase in PaCO$_2$ (PaCO$_2$ >6.7 kPa (50.2mmHg), it is described as type II respiratory failure (Burns 2014).

PaO$_2$ is a major factor in determining SaO$_2$, or the affinity of haemoglobin to oxygen, and this relationship is often demonstrated by the oxyhaemoglobin dissociation curve (Lian 2010).

Table 2.1 Oxygen saturation and partial pressure of oxygen levels

	Normal	Less than normal
SaO_2	92–98%	Hypoxemia
PaO_2	>10.6kPa	Hypoxemia

Step 3: Assess the pH

Assessment of the pH will determine whether there is alkalemia or acidemia present, and thus usually identifies the primary cause of the ABG abnormality.

Please note: Acidosis and alkalosis can be present even if the pH is within the normal range; and $PaCO_2$, HCO_3^- and anion gap must be taken into account.

pH

Potential hydrogen (pH) determines the concentration of hydrogen ions (H^+) found in arterial blood. The normal pH value of arterial blood is between 7.34 and 7.45mmol/l, and is maintained by a balance between the alkalis and the acids in the body. There is an inverse proportional relationship between the pH and H^+ concentrations: a fall in pH results in a rise in H^+ concentration, indicating acidemia; while a rise in pH results in a fall of H^+ concentration, indicating alkalemia (Lian 2010).

Table 2.2 Normal and abnormal pH levels

	Normal	Less than normal	Greater than normal
pH	7.35–7.45	Acidosis	Alkalosis

The more acidotic the blood becomes (with a pH of less than 7.35), the more the force of cardiac contraction and the vascular response to catecholamine decrease. The body also becomes less responsive to the effects of certain medications. (Coombs 2001). On the other hand, when blood becomes alkalotic (with a pH of more than 7.35), there is interference with tissue oxygenation, as well as neurological functioning, and muscular performance is affected (Coombs 2001). If these changes in pH remain uncorrected (so that the pH is greater than 7.8 or lower than 6.8), this will result in cells dying, due to the significant impact on cellular functioning (Orlando Health Education and Development 2010). In order to maintain homeostasis and keep the pH within normal limits, the respiratory system, the renal system, and the buffer system work to eliminate or produce H^+ (acid) and bicarbonate (alkaline).

Step 4: Assess for respiratory disturbance

A respiratory disturbance is determined by the direction of change in the pH to that of the $PaCO_2$.

PaCO$_2$

The partial pressure of carbon dioxide (PaCO$_2$) is the measurement of the carbon dioxide dissolved in the blood, which reflects alveolar ventilation (Singh *et al.* 2013). Normal PaCO$_2$ of arterial blood is 4.5−6 kilopascal (kPa) (33.7−45mmHg). Therefore, as a rule, if the pH and the PaCO$_2$ change in opposite directions, the primary disorder is respiratory.

CO$_2$, a waste product of cellular metabolism, is carried by the blood and eliminated via the lungs. This process is regulated by the respiratory centre in the brain, which controls the rate and depth of breathing and therefore determines the amount of CO$_2$ the body needs to exhale, to maintain adequate pH levels. An accumulation of CO$_2$ in the body, due to alveolar hypoventilation, increases the acidity of the blood and causes the pH to decrease (Singh *et al.* 2013). Similarly, if there were a decrease in CO$_2$, due to hyperventilation, this would increase the alkalinity of the blood, causing the pH to increase (Singh *et al.* 2013).

Table 2.3 Normal and abnormal partial pressure of carbon dioxide

Normal	Less than normal	Greater than normal	
PaCO2	4.5–6kPa (33.7–45mmHg)	Alkalosis	Acidosis

Step 5: Assess for metabolic disturbance

A metabolic disturbance is determined by the direction of the pH to that of the HCO3-.

HCO$_3^-$

Bicarbonate (HCO$_3$) is the metabolic component in an ABG and represents the concentration of hydrogen carbonate in the blood. The normal level of HCO$_3^-$ in the blood is 22−26mmol. As a rule, if the HCO$_3^-$ and the pH changes in the same direction, the primary disorder is of a metabolic component (Singh *et al.* 2013).

HCO3$^-$ is a base that is regulated by the kidneys (Singh *et al.* 2013) and is the main chemical buffer in plasma. Some metabolic disorders can cause an increase in circulatory acids, or loss of the HCO$_3^-$ (base) in the body. This leads to a decrease in blood pH (i.e. acidosis), while the body makes efforts to retain HCO$_3^-$. Likewise, if there is an increase in HCO$_3^-$ or a loss of metabolic acids within the body, the pH will increase (alkalosis), as the body tries to excrete HCO$_3^-$ via the urine.

Base excess (BE)

Base excess is another measure used to determine the metabolic component of an acid-base disturbance, and all bases (including bicarbonate) are measured. The base excess is described as the amount of acid (or hydrogen ions) required to correct the pH of the blood to a normal range. It is calculated using blood pH and PaCO$_2$. The normal range for base excess is between -2 and +2mmol per litre of blood. However, this can increase in metabolic alkalosis, and can decrease in metabolic acidosis (Verma & Roach 2010).

BE is a calculated value, and should not be used in isolation to determine metabolic disturbances. However, it can be used with HCO_3, as having a high BE is the same as having a high HCO_3 (Burns 2014).

Anion gap

When used with other investigations (such as lactate, creatinine, plasma glucose and urine ketone), the anion gap (AG) can diagnose the presence of metabolic acidosis. It can also differentiate the causes and the severity of the disturbance, as well as measuring the responses to treatment. The AG represents the difference between cations (positively charged ions such as Na^+ and K^+) and anions (negatively charged ions such as Cl^- and HCO_3) in the body, and is calculated using the following formula:

$$Anion\ gap = Na^+ - (Cl^- + HCO_3^-)$$

The normal value for the AG is $8-16$mmol. A decrease in the AG is often caused by hypoalbuminemia, severe haemodilution or inaccurate lab results, while diarrhoea and loss of urinary bicarbonates can have a normal anion gap. Dehydration or increases in minor ions (such as ketones and lactate) can cause an increase in anion gap (Verma & Roach 2010).

Table 2.4 Normal and abnormal bicarbonate, base excess and anion gap

	Normal	Less than normal	Greater than normal
HCO_3	22–26	Acidosis	Alkalosis
BE	-2 to +2	Acidosis	Alkalosis
AG	12 +/-4	Acidosis	Alkalosis

Step 6: Establish if the disturbance is compensatory or mixed

Compensatory disturbance

Once the primary acid-base disorder is identified as the cause of the acid-base disturbance, the compensatory system attempts to return the pH back to normal by altering its buffering system. For example, if the problem is a respiratory abnormality, the kidneys (or the metabolic system) will regulate the amount of hydrogen ion and HCO_3 that is eliminated or absorbed, and compensation can occur over two to five days. In contrast, for metabolic abnormalities, the respiratory system will compensate by altering CO_2 excretion. It does this by adjusting respiratory pattern, rate and depth, and compensation can occur over a period ranging between 12 and 24 hours. The degree to which compensation is (or is not) occurring also needs to be established, as an ABG can be partially compensated (with the pH approaching the normal range) or fully compensated (with the pH in normal range).

Mixed disturbances

When compensatory mechanisms have returned the pH to normal range, a mixed disturbance (a combination of two or more primary aetiologies) is suspected. A mixed disturbance makes it difficult to match the ABG with expected values of acidosis, alkalosis and the compensatory response. The treatment of mixed disorders is geared towards correcting the acid-base disturbances involved. Some examples of mixed disturbances are:

- Mixed metabolic disorders, such as lactic acidosis and diabetic ketone acidosis
- Mixed respiratory-metabolic disorders, such as respiratory acidosis and metabolic acidosis, or respiratory acidosis and metabolic alkalosis or respiratory alkalosis and metabolic acidosis.

Please note: It is not possible to have mixed respiratory disorders (such as respiratory acidosis and respiratory alkalosis) at the same time.

Conclusion

In summary, the following six-step approach can be used to interpret ABGs.

Table 2.5 Six-step approach to ABG interpretation

Step 1: Review the patient   Examine the patient for clues as to the type of disturbance.
Step 2: Analyse the oxygenation   Look for signs of hypoxia, by assessing the PaO_2 and SaO_2.
Step 3: Assess the pH   Determine the acid balance. Check the pH for acidemia or alkalemia.
Step 4: Assess for respiratory disturbance   Consider the state of alveolar ventilation by evaluating the $PaCO_2$.
Step 5: Assess for metabolic disturbance   Examine HCO_3^- and BE in relation to pH, to determine metabolic involvement.
Step 6: Establish if the disturbance is compensatory or mixed   Observe the pH to determine if the compensation is appropriate for the primary disturbance (i.e. complete or partial).

References

Burns, G. (2014). Arterial blood gases made easy. *Clinical Medicine.* **14**(1), 66–68.

Coombs, M. (2001). *Making sense of arterial blood gases.* http://www.nursingtimes.net/clinical-archive/haematology/making-sense-of-arterial-blood-gases/200822.fullarticle (accessed 2 July 2016).

Lian, J.X. (2010). Interpreting and using the arterial blood gas analysis. *Nursing2010 Critical Care.* **5**(3), 26–36.

Lynch, F. (2009). Arterial blood gas analysis: Implications for Nursing. *Paediatric Nurse.* **21**(1), 41–44.

Orlando Health, Education & Development (2010). *Interpretation of Arterial Blood Gases. Self-Learning Packet.* https://www.coursehero.com/file/11324678/ABG-self-learning/ (accessed 2 July 2016).

Singh, V., Khatana, K. & Gupta, P. (2013). Blood gas analysis for bedside diagnosis. *National Journal of Maxillofacial Surgery.* **4**(2), 136–41.

Verma, A.K. & Roach, P. (2010). The interpretation of arterial blood gases. *Australian Prescriber.* **33**, 124–29.

3

Respiratory acidosis

Dawn Parsons

Respiratory acidosis is a disruption in acid-base balance caused by alveolar hypoventilation. Carbon dioxide is produced rapidly, and failure of ventilation increases the partial pressure of arterial carbon dioxide ($PaCO_2$) (Byrd et al. 2015).

Alveolar hypoventilation leads to an increased $PaCO_2$ (hypercapnia). The increase in $PaCO_2$ decreases the bicarbonate (HCO_3^-)/$PaCO_2$ ratio, which in turn decreases the pH. When ventilation is impaired and the respiratory system removes less carbon dioxide than the amount produced in the tissues, hypercapnia and respiratory acidosis result.

Weatherspoon (2015) indicates that there are two forms of respiratory acidosis: acute and chronic. Acute respiratory acidosis is rapid in onset; it is considered an emergency situation and can become life-threatening if not managed. In contrast, chronic respiratory acidosis develops over a period of time and is asymptomatic. Over time, the body adapts to the increased acidity. However, this chapter will focus on acute respiratory acidosis.

Causes of hypoventilation and respiratory acidosis

Respiratory acidosis is most frequently caused by a lung disease or by a condition that affects normal breathing or impairs the lung's ability to remove CO_2.

Lung disorder causes include:

- Emphysema
- Chronic bronchitis
- Severe asthma
- Pneumonia
- Pneumothorax.

Neuromuscular causes include:

- Diaphragm dysfunction and paralysis
- Guillain-Barré Syndrome

- Myasthenia Gravis
- Muscular dystrophy
- Motor neurone disease.

Chest wall causes include:

- Severe kyphoscoliosis
- Status post thoracoplasty
- Flail chest.

Central nervous system (CNS) depression causes include:

- Drugs (e.g. narcotics, barbiturates, benzodiazepines, and other CNS depressants).

Neurologic causes include:

- Encephalitis
- Brainstem disease and trauma
- Brain tumour or abscess.

Other causes include:

- Obesity-hypoventilation syndrome
- Obstructive sleep apnoea
- Lung-protective mechanical ventilation with permissive hypercapnia in the treatment of acute respiratory distress syndrome (ARDS).

Presenting signs and symptoms of respiratory acidosis

Clinical signs and symptoms of respiratory acidosis are often varied and are those related to the underlying disorder. They are dependent on the severity of the disorder and on the rate of development of hypercapnia. Slow-developing mild to moderate hypercapnia usually has minimal symptoms. As the partial arterial pressure of carbon dioxide ($PaCO_2$) increases, anxiety may progress to delirium and patients become progressively more confused, drowsy and eventually impossible to rouse.

Treatment of respiratory acidosis

Treating acute respiratory acidosis is primarily focused on addressing the underlying disorder or pathophysiologic process. This must be done as soon as possible and artificial ventilation may also be required to manage this. The criteria for admission to the intensive care unit (ICU) varies between regions, but may include patient confusion, lethargy, respiratory muscle fatigue, and a low pH (<7.25). Any patient who requires tracheal intubation and mechanical ventilation must be admitted to the ICU.

Some acute care facilities require patients being treated acutely with non-invasive positive-pressure ventilation (NIPPV) to be admitted to the ICU or high dependency unit (HDU). Past medical history, presenting symptoms, physical examination, and any available results following investigations, should be used to guide the patient's treatment. The treatment may also include: bronchodilators to reverse some types of airway obstruction, antibiotics, oxygen therapy to reduce hypoxia, and non-invasive positive-pressure ventilation (sometimes called CPAP or BiPAP).

Case study 3.1

Patient C, a 38-year-old woman, returned to the gynaecological ward following a total abdominal hysterectomy for fibroids and menorrhagia. The surgical procedure was performed under general anaesthetic with intravenous paracetamol, morphine sulphate and diclofenac per rectum administered for intra-operative analgesia. Intravenous cyclizine was also administered for its anti-emetic property (BNF 2015). Patient C experienced high levels of postoperative pain in the recovery unit and was administered bolus doses of morphine sulphate via a prescribed patient-controlled analgesia (PCA) before returning to the ward.

On return to the ward, the patient was drowsy, but rousable and described her pain as 4 out of 10 on a numerical rating score. Intravenous fluid was in progress alongside the PCA and the patient had a urinary catheter in situ, which was patent and draining. Patient C's clinical parameters were within normal limits on return to the ward. Her observations were as follows: blood pressure 118/78; heart rate 74bpm; SpO_2 99% on 2Lpm of oxygen via nasal specs; respiratory rate of 9 per minute; and a temperature of 36.8°C.

An hour later, Patient C's husband reported to the nurse in charge that he was worried about his wife and that she was no longer answering him and didn't appear to be breathing.

Case study 3.1: Assessment and treatment

The systematic ABCDE approach to patient assessment will be used, as indicated by the Resuscitation Council (2015). This includes assessment of the **A**irway, **B**reathing, **C**irculation, **D**isability and **E**xposure. This approach enables the practitioner to identify and treat life-threatening issues as a priority and assess the effectiveness of any treatment.

Airway: Patient C was demonstrating evidence of airway obstruction with audible snoring noises, requiring an oral pharyngeal airway. At this point the medical team were called to attend.

Breathing: On examination she had bilateral air entry, demonstrating no use of accessory muscles, and was bradypnoeic with a respiratory rate of 5. There was no audible wheeze noted and her SpO_2 was 99% on 2Lpm. As this was an emergency situation, oxygen therapy was commenced on high flow via a non-rebreathe oxygen mask. An arterial blood gas (ABG) was taken, resulting in a pH of 7.25; $PaCO_2$ of 8.2 (61.5mmHg); and HCO_3 of 21. This ABG demonstrates respiratory acidosis, due to her pH being low, $PaCO_2$ being high and a low HCO_3.

Circulation: Patient C had a blood pressure recorded at 88/42, with a tachycardia of 102 and a temperature recorded at 36.6°C. Her colour was pink and she appeared well perfused. A 12-lead echocardiogram (ECG) demonstrated sinus tachycardia with nil else noted. Patient C also had a capillary refill time assessed as <2. Intravenous Hartman's continued to run, as prescribed.

Disability: A rapid assessment of Patient C's conscious level was performed using the AVPU method: **A**lert, responds to **V**oice, responds to **P**ain or is **U**nresponsive to all stimuli (Resuscitation Council 2014–2016). She demonstrated no evidence of response to stimuli and was therefore assessed as unresponsive, which was also consistent with her inability to protect her own airway. On assessment, her pupils were of an equal size and were reactive to light, but were pin point in size, which can be indicative of opiate overdose. This was also a potential consideration due to her low blood pressure and tachycardia. Her blood sugar was normal at 5.5mmol/l.

Patient C had received a large amount of morphine intra-operatively, postoperatively and on return to the ward by using the patient-controlled handset. The medical team considered that this accumulation of morphine had caused low blood pressure, high heart rate and hypoventilation, thus leading to respiratory acidosis and the resulting unresponsiveness.

An antagonist was therefore prescribed, in the form of naloxone (BNF 2015) to reverse the effects of the morphine. However, it must be noted that reversing the morphine can potentially also reverse the analgesic effect required for the surgical procedure. Naloxone also has a short half-life so the patient must be continually monitored for further deterioration (Clark et al. 2005). Administering a morphine antagonist will increase respiratory rate, increase blood pressure and reduce heart rate, which will in turn increase the patient's pH and reduce their $PaCO_2$. This will also reverse respiratory acidosis, thus enhancing alertness.

Patient C required admission to the ICU for intubation and ventilation for several hours to assist in regulating her respiratory rate and therefore reduce her $PaCO_2$. As soon as the naloxone was administered, an increase in respiratory rate was noted. However, after an hour or so, she would metabolise the antagonist and her respiratory rate would drop again.

Exposure: On exposure of Patient C, her wound demonstrated minimal ooze and her per vaginal loss was also minimal, with nil else of note.

Six-step ABG interpretation of case study 3.1

Step 1: Review the patient
Given the information in the above scenario, this patient displayed physical signs and symptoms of hypoventilation due to the high administration and accumulation of postoperative opioids.
Step 2: Analyse the oxygenation
The O_2 and SaO_2 are within the normal range.
Step 3: Assess the pH
The pH indicates acidemia.

Step 4: Assess for respiratory disturbance The pCO_2 is high, and goes in the opposite direction to the pH; the primary problem is therefore respiratory.
Step 5: Assess for metabolic disturbance The HCO_3 and BE are normal.
Step 6: Establish if the disturbance is compensatory or mixed N/A
Interpretation: Respiratory acidosis.

It has been established that this patient displayed physical signs and symptoms of hypoventilation, with physiological evidence of respiratory acidosis that was gained from an ABG. The hypoventilation experienced was due to the high administration and accumulation of postoperative opioids. Due to prompt assessment, investigation and treatment, the symptoms were managed effectively. Discontinuing the patient's PCA and administering high-flow oxygen, naloxone, intubation and ventilation for a short period enabled healthcare staff to reverse the respiratory acidosis. This allowed the patient's clinical parameters to return to normal limits, and she could then be discharged to the ward before being sent home (on alternative analgesia) several days later.

Case study 3.2

Patient D, a 71-year-old woman, lives alone in a bungalow with her cat. She suffers from osteoarthritis and is on the waiting list for a total hip replacement. She takes regular paracetamol and oral morphine sulphate for pain; otherwise she is well for her age. Patient D has recently had a bad cold. However, over the last eight days, she has been feeling generally unwell and finding it difficult to catch her breath. She has been feeling fatigued and has lost her appetite, which is normally very good. She has been referred to the medical ward by her GP with an audible wheeze, dyspnoea, pyrexia and chest pain on inspiration.

Case study 3.2: Assessment and treatment

Airway: Patient D was unable to talk in sentences due to her shortness of breath. This provided evidence of a patent airway and no airway obstruction.

Breathing: On examination, Patient D had equal air entry, was using accessory muscles and was tachyphnoeic with a respiratory rate of 34. She was also noted to have a cough and her SpO_2 was 87% on air. As it was an emergency situation, oxygen therapy was initially commenced on high flow via a non-rebreathe oxygen mask. An arterial blood gas (ABG) was taken, resulting in a pH of 7.20, $PaCO_2$ of 8.8 (66mmHg), HCO_3 of 20 and PaO_2 of 9.8 (73.5mmHg). This ABG demonstrates respiratory acidosis, due to the pH being low, $PaCO_2$ being high, low PaO_2 demonstrating hypoxia and a low HCO_3.

Patients who are hypoxaemic and hypercapnic are considered to be in respiratory failure type 2 (Nair & Peate 2009). For this patient, the aim of the treatment was to improve ventilation. This involved commencing non-invasive positive pressure ventilation (NIPPV), which increased depth of breathing so that the patient was able to blow off $PaCO_2$ effectively. A chest x-ray was also performed, leading to a diagnosis of pneumonia, with right lower lobe consolidation. A broad-spectrum intravenous antibiotic was prescribed, prior to receiving a sputum test result.

Circulation: Patient D's blood pressure was recorded at 94/42, with a tachycardia of 130 and a temperature recorded at 38.9°C. Routine bloods confirmed an elevated white blood cell count and C-reactive protein, indicating infection (Leach 2012). Her face was flushed, but her lips appeared slightly cyanosed. A 12-lead echocardiogram (ECG) demonstrated sinus tachycardia with nil else noted. Patient D also had a capillary refill time assessed as >3. Intravenous fluids were administered, as prescribed to rehydrate the patient. Physiotherapy was also initiated to aid sputum clearance. An upright patient position is essential to enhance diaphragm and intercostal muscle activity and therefore improve ventilation.

Disability: Patient D was awake, but slightly confused on admission to the ward. Her blood sugar was normal at 4.4mmol/l. When the patient's chest pain was assessed, it was worse on inspiration and expiration (pleuritic in nature) and scored 5 out of 10 on a numerical rating score, indicating mild to moderate pain. She had already taken her regular paracetamol (which would help reduce her pyrexia) and oral morphine as prescribed for her chronic osteoarthritis. A further dose of an oral opiate was administered in order to reduce the pain experienced and encourage effective breathing and coughing. Nausea was not experienced, but an anti-emetic was prescribed as a prophylactic measure.

Exposure: During exposure of the patient, the patient's skin was noted to be hot, clammy and flushed. Nil else was noted.

Six-step ABG interpretation of case study 3.2

Step 1: Review the patient Given the information in the above scenario, this patient displayed physical signs and symptoms of pneumonia. Pneumonia disrupts external respiration and less oxygen diffuses from the alveoli into the pulmonary circulation, thus causing hypercapnia and hypoxia.
Step 2: Analyse the oxygenation The O_2 and SaO_2 are low. Oxygen therapy commenced.
Step 3: Assess the pH The pH indicates acidemia.
Step 4: Assess for respiratory disturbance The pCO_2 is high, and goes in the opposite direction to the pH; the primary problem is therefore respiratory.
Step 5: Assess for metabolic disturbance The HCO_3 and BE are normal.

Step 6: Establish if the disturbance is Compensatory or Mixed
N/A
Interpretation:
Respiratory acidosis.

It has been established that this patient displayed physical signs and symptoms of pneumonia, with an ABG that confirmed respiratory acidosis. Pneumonia with consolidation in the alveoli disrupts external respiration. Less oxygen diffuses from the alveoli into the pulmonary circulation, thus causing hypercapnia, hypoxia and therefore respiratory acidosis. With prompt assessment, investigation and treatment, symptoms were managed effectively with NIPPV, antibiotics, physiotherapy, Intravenous fluids and effective analgesia. Patient D received care in the HDU for several days and returned to a medical ward, once the acute episode of respiratory acidosis was resolved and her clinical parameters were returning to within normal limits.

References

Byrd, R. (2015). *Respiratory Alkalosis*. http://emedicine.medscape.com/article/301680-overview (accessed 24 June 2016).

British National Formulary (BNF) (2015). BNF Publications. http://www.bnf.org/ (accessed 4 July 2016).

Clark, J., Dargan, P. & Jones, A. (2005). Naloxone in opioid poisoning: walking the tightrope. *Emergency Medicine*. **22**, 612–16.

Leach, R. (2012). *Acute and Critical Care Medicine at a Glance*. 2nd edn. Chichester: Wiley & Sons Ltd.

Nair, M. & Peate, I. (2009). *Fundamentals of Applied Pathophysiology: An essential guide for nursing students*. 1st edn. Chichester: Wiley & Sons.

National Institute for Health and Care Excellence (NICE) (2012). *Pulmonary embolism: Managing confirmed pulmonary embolism*. http://cks.nice.org.uk/pulmonary-embolism#!scenario:1 (accessed 24 June 2016).

Resuscitation Council (2014–2016). *Guidelines and guidance, The ABCDE Approach, Underlying principles*. https://www.resus.org.uk/resuscitation-guidelines/abcde-approach/ (accessed 24 June 2016).

Weatherspoon, D. (2015). *Respiratory Acidosis*. http://www.healthline.com/health/respiratory-acidosis#Overview1 (accessed 4 July 2016).

4

Respiratory alkalosis
Dawn Parsons

Respiratory alkalosis is the disruption of acid-base balance due to alveolar hyperventilation, leading to reduced partial pressure of arterial carbon dioxide ($PaCO_2$). The reduced $PaCO_2$ increases the ratio of bicarbonate concentration and therefore elevates the blood pH. The reduction in $PaCO_2$ (hypocapnia) develops when a robust respiratory stimulus causes the respiratory system to remove more carbon dioxide than is produced metabolically in the tissues (Byrd 2015).

The normal range for $PaCO_2$ is 4.5–6 kPa (33.7–45mmHg). When the chemoreceptors in the brain and carotid bodies sense hydrogen concentrations, they influence ventilation to adjust the $PaCO_2$ and pH. When these receptors sense an increase in hydrogen ions, respiration is increased to 'blow off' the carbon dioxide and reduce the hydrogen ions. However, disease processes can increase ventilation, with increasing hyperventilation leading to hypocapnia.

In acute onset of respiratory alkalosis, the $PaCO_2$ level falls below the minimum level of normal and the blood pH becomes alkalemic. In chronic respiratory alkalosis, the $PaCO_2$ level falls below the minimum limit of normal, but the pH is near normal or normal.

Causes of hyperventilation and respiratory alkalosis

Hyperventilation due to a panic attack is the most common cause of respiratory alkalosis, which is often known as over-breathing and results from rapid or heavy breathing. Although this is the primary cause of respiratory alkalosis, there are other potential causes, which are listed below.

Central nervous system causes include:

- Head injury
- Cardiovascular accident (CVA)
- Anxiety (hyperventilation syndrome)
- Supra-tentorial (e.g. pain, fear, stress)
- Pyrexia
- Chronic liver failure

- Drug induced (e.g. salicylate intoxication, aminophyllines)
- Endogenous compounds (e.g. progesterone during pregnancy, cytokines during sepsis).

Hypoxemia or tissue hypoxia causes include:

- High altitude
- Respiratory stimulation via peripheral chemoreceptors.

Pulmonary causes include:

- Pulmonary embolism
- Pneumonia
- Asthma
- Pulmonary oedema
- Chronic obstructive pulmonary disease (COPD).

Cardiac causes include:

- Myocardial infarction.

Iatrogenic causes include:

- Excessive controlled ventilation.

Presenting signs and symptoms of respiratory alkalosis

The clinical signs and symptoms of respiratory alkalosis depend on the duration and severity of the underlying cause or disease process. Hyperventilation is in itself an indication that respiratory alkalosis may develop. However, in acute episodes hypocapnia can lead to cerebral vasoconstriction, reducing cerebral blood flow and resulting in neurologic symptoms including: dizziness, light-headedness, dry mouth, confusion, numbness in extremities and lips, syncope and seizures. However, there are also some signs and symptoms that are unrelated to the change in pH. Chest tightness, dyspnoea and headache may also be noted in psychogenic hyperventilation, along with other symptoms unrelated to alkalemia but potentially related to anxiety.

Treatment of respiratory alkalosis

Treatment for respiratory alkalosis is mainly focused on resolving the underlying cause, which involves elevation of blood CO_2. Treatment may therefore include several management strategies aimed at reducing blood CO_2. Some strategies may involve oxygen therapy, reassurance, rebreathing into a paper bag, diuretics and breath-holding techniques. Alternatively, if the patient is intubated, reduction of minute volume ventilation is required by adjusting the rate and tidal volume. Other methods could include using a 'Sigh' function or positive end expiratory pressure (PEEP) to hold the inspiratory phase a little longer.

In order to apply theory to practice and understand patient presentation, assessment, treatment and management, two case studies will be presented.

Case study 4.1

Patient A is a 54-year-old woman who has been admitted to accident and emergency following a fall from her bicycle. She has sustained an injury to her right wrist, with obvious abnormality. Patient A suffers from anxiety attacks, which have become worse following a significant family bereavement. When the paramedic team arrived at the scene they found her confused, shaken, distressed with pain and breathless. She was complaining of pain in her wrist and being unable to catch her breath. She was also experiencing numbness in her lips, and pins and needles in her fingers.

Case study 4.1: Assessment and treatment

The systematic ABCDE approach to patient assessment will be used, as indicated by the Resuscitation Council (2015). This includes assessment of the **A**irway, **B**reathing, **C**irculation, **D**isability and **E**xposure. This approach enables the practitioner to identify and treat life-threatening issues as a priority and assess the effectiveness of any treatment.

Airway: The patient was talking, although confused, providing evidence that her airway was patent with no signs of airway obstruction.

Breathing: She had bilateral air entry with no audible wheeze present, she was tachyphnoeic with a respiratory rate of 36 per minute and her SpO_2 was 99% on air. An arterial blood gas (ABG) was taken, resulting in a pH of 7.46, $PaCO_2$ of 4.5 (33.7mmHg) and HCO_3 of 26. This ABG demonstrates respiratory alkalosis, due to her pH being elevated, $PaCO_2$ being low and a normal HCO_3.

At this point, Patient A was encouraged to try to slow her breathing and was given a paper bag to breathe into. This encouraged the rebreathing of her own carbon dioxide, which allowed her $PaCO_2$ levels to rise within normal limits and thereby reduced her respiratory rate. However, rebreathing via a paper bag must be used with caution if there is an uncertain diagnosis or if the patient has comorbidities. Continual encouragement was required for Patient A to adapt her breathing techniques until the pain began to reduce.

Circulation: Patient A had an intravenous cannula sited. This was done in order to obtain baseline bloods and in case surgery was required. Her blood pressure was 185/102, with a heart rate of 105 and a temperature recorded at 36.6°C. It could be suggested that the hypertension and tachycardia was related to the pain experienced due to the displaced wrist injury.

Disability: Patient A was rousable when a neurological assessment was performed. Her blood sugar was normal, at 4.8mmol/l. The patient's pain was assessed, and scored at 8 out of 10, using a numerical rating score, and she was noted to be in severe acute pain. This pain was treated with a multimodal approach to analgesia, using paracetamol, a non-steroidal anti-inflammatory and an intravenous opiate in increments until the pain score reduced, with evidence of her physiological symptoms also settling. No nausea was experienced.

Exposure: No injuries were noted during exposure of the patient, except for a significant displacement of the right wrist. An x-ray was performed, demonstrating a distal ulna and radial fracture, which required surgery.

Six-step ABG interpretation of case study 4.1

Step 1: Review the patient Given the information in the above scenario, this patient displayed physical signs and symptoms of hyperventilation. This was not only due to her history of anxiety attacks, but also the severe pain experienced from the wrist injury, which caused her to become tachypneic, tachycardic and hypertensive.
Step 2: Analyse the oxygenation The O_2 and SaO_2 are within range.
Step 3: Assess the pH The pH indicates alkalemia.
Step 4: Assess for respiratory disturbance The pCO_2 is low, and goes in the opposite direction to the pH; the primary problem is therefore respiratory.
Step 5: Assess for metabolic disturbance The HCO_3 and BE are normal.
Step 6: Establish if the disturbance is compensatory or mixed N/A
Interpretation: Respiratory alkalosis.

It has been established that this patient displayed physical signs and symptoms of hyperventilation. Physiological evidence of respiratory alkalosis was gained from an ABG. Her hyperventilation could possibly have been due to the combination of an anxiety attack and the severe pain experienced from her wrist injury, causing her to become tachypnoeic, tachycardic and hypertensive. With prompt assessment of her arterial blood gas, treatment was initiated to reduce her respiratory rate, retaining more PCO_2, thus returning it to normal and reducing the signs and symptoms experienced. Effective analgesia was also administered, which reduced the pain, resulting in the patient's blood pressure, respiratory and heart rate returning to within normal limits. The patient received surgical care and returned home the following day with advice and education on breathing exercises to carry out during an anxiety attack.

Case study 4.2

Patient B was a 48-year-old man with a body mass index (BMI) of 36. He was on a surgical ward, recovering from a Hartman's procedure for a perforated diverticulitis. He was a fairly heavy smoker (25 per day) and enjoyed drinking socially at weekends. There was nil of note in his past medical history. He was not on any prescribed medication and worked as a foreman on a building site.

On day 4 of his postoperative recovery, he complained of sudden onset of chest pain and shortness of breath on returning to his bed from the bathroom.

Case study 4.2: Assessment and treatment

Airway: Patient B was able to talk, although he was struggling to string a sentence together. This provided evidence of a patent airway and no sign of airway obstruction. At this point the medical team were called to attend.

Breathing: On examination, he had bilateral air entry, was using accessory muscles and was tachyphnoeic with a respiratory rate of 25. There was no audible wheeze noted and his SpO_2 was 91% on air. As this was an emergency situation, oxygen therapy was commenced on high flow via a non-rebreathe oxygen mask. An arterial blood gas (ABG) was taken, resulting in a pH of 7.5, $PaCO_2$ of 4.2 (31.5mmHg) and HCO_3 of 27. This ABG demonstrates respiratory alkalosis, due to his pH being elevated, $PaCO_2$ being low and a slightly elevated HCO_3.

Circulation: Patient B had a blood pressure recorded at 98/46, with a tachycardia of 102 and a temperature recorded at 36.6°C. He appeared pale, clammy and his lips were slightly cyanosed, demonstrating signs of hypoxia. A 12-lead echocardiogram demonstrated sinus tachycardia and very slight ST segment changes. Patient B also had a capillary refill time assessed as 3. Intravenous normal saline was initiated to compensate for poor fluid tissue perfusion.

Disability: Patient B was rousable when a neurological assessment was performed. His blood sugar was normal at 6.8mmol/l. The patient's chest pain was assessed, and scored as 6 out of 10, using a numerical rating score, and he was noted to be in moderate pain. He was already receiving regular analgesia for his surgical procedure, so an intravenous opiate was administered and reviewed regularly until his physiological symptoms of pain started settling. Nausea was experienced and therefore an anti-emetic (50mg cyclizine) was administered as prescribed.

Exposure: No abnormalities were noted during exposure, until Patient B's left calf was examined. On examination, he complained of discomfort in his calf, which was slightly swollen and red. This immediately led the medical team to consider a deep vein thrombosis (DVT), leading to a pulmonary embolism (PE). This initiated various investigations, including a chest X-ray which demonstrated no abnormalities. A Doppler ultrasound sonography confirmed a lower leg DVT and a D-dimer test proved positive for a thrombus. A V/Q scan was then performed. This confirmed a high probability of a PE, along with high clinical suspicion, which Leach (2012) indicates has a positive predictive value of >95%.

According to the National Institute for Health and Care Excellence (2012) parenteral anticoagulants are recommended in the initial phase of pulmonary embolism treatment to ensure rapid anti-coagulation, to reduce the risk of harm from thrombosis propagation or further embolic events.

Six-step ABG interpretation of case study 4.2

Step 1: Review the patient
Given the information in the above scenario, Patient B displayed physical signs and symptoms of hyperventilation due to the acute episode of shortness of breath caused by a pulmonary embolism.
Step 2: Analyse the oxygenation
The O_2 and SaO_2 levels are below the normal range so oxygen therapy is commenced.
Step 3: Assess the pH
The pH indicates alkalemia.
Step 4: Assess for respiratory disturbance
The pCO_2 is low, and goes in the opposite direction to the pH; the primary problem is therefore respiratory.
Step 5: Assess for metabolic disturbance
The HCO_3 and BE are normal.
Step 6: Establish if the disturbance is compensatory or mixed
N/A
Interpretation:
Respiratory alkalosis.

It has been established that this patient displayed physical signs and symptoms of hyperventilation with physiological evidence of respiratory alkalosis, gained from an ABG. The hyperventilation experienced was due to the acute episode of shortness of breath caused by a pulmonary embolism. With prompt assessment, investigation and treatment, his symptoms were managed effectively. The administration of intravenous fluids, analgesia, anti-emetic, high-flow oxygen and anticoagulant therapy (during an acute episode) allowed the patient to return home several days later, with ongoing anti-coagulation therapy and education around lifestyle changes.

References

Byrd, R. (2015). *Respiratory Alkalosis.* http://emedicine.medscape.com/article/301680-overview (accessed 27 June 2016).

Leach, R. (2012). *Acute and Critical Care Medicine at a Glance.* 2nd edn. Chichester: Wiley & Sons Ltd.

National Institute for Health and Care Excellence (NICE) (2012). *Pulmonary Embolism: Managing confirmed pulmonary embolism.* http://cks.nice.org.uk/pulmonary-embolism#!scenario:1 (accessed 27 June 2016).

Resuscitation Council (2015). *Guidelines and guidance, The ABCDE Approach, Underlying principles.* https://www.resus.org.uk/resuscitation-guidelines/abcde-approach/ (accessed 27 June 2016).

5

Metabolic acidosis

Stanley Swanepoel

This chapter will look at the presentation, identification and management of metabolic acidosis, which is commonly seen in the perioperative environment. The scenario is fictitious but does resemble expected findings in clinical practice.

Causes of metabolic acidosis

The most common cause of metabolic acidosis is an increase in the production of fixed or organic acids, which causes a fall in the pH of the blood. This is the bicarbonate buffer system, which may be influenced by three main factors:

- Lactic acidosis
- Ketoacidosis
- Severe loss of bicarbonate.

Lactic acidosis

This is usually a result of either strenuous exercise or tissue hypoxia, caused by anaerobic respiration within the cells.

Ketoacidosis

Ketoacidosis can arise as a result of starvation or poorly controlled diabetes mellitus. Impaired hydrogen (H^+) secretion by the kidneys (due to kidney damage) is a less frequent cause. Diuretics that turn off the sodium–hydrogen transport system in the kidney tubules can also lead to metabolic acidosis. This occurs because the secretion of H^+ is linked to the reabsorption of sodium (Na^+). When the reabsorption of sodium stops, the secretion of H^+ stops.

Severe loss of bicarbonate

This is the third factor influencing metabolic acidosis. Bicarbonate ions are used to balance hydrogen ions in the carbonic acid–bicarbonate buffering system and thus maintain the pH balance within the body. Pancreatic, hepatic and mucosal secretions are relied upon to carry the carbonate ions into the bowel. These ions are then reabsorbed before the faeces are eliminated. When a patient has chronic diarrhoea, this reabsorption does not take place, with a resulting loss of carbonate and a subsequent reduction in the HCO_3.

Case study 5.1

A 58-year-old man was admitted to the emergency department with suspected aortic aneurysm. He was normally fit and well, with mild hypertension.

It was determined that emergency surgical intervention was required and he was prepared for emergency admission to the operating theatre.

The patient received a general anaesthetic with positive pressure ventilation and radial artery arterial line. Two large-bore peripheral cannulas, a urinary catheter and a central venous cannula were all inserted prior to surgery. The patient was warmed with external warm air heating blankets and intravenous fluid warmers. At this stage the patient's blood gases were within normal ranges and his haemoglobin level was 14g/dl. As the surgery progressed, cross-clamping of the aorta took place at the infra-renal level, to enable the repair of the aneurysm.

Case study 5.1: Assessment and treatment

At the time of cross-clamping, an arterial blood gas sample was sent off and the results were: a pH of 7.4, pCO_2 of 5.33 (39.9mmHg), pO_2 of 13.1 (98.2mmHg), HCO_3 of 24, and BE of 0.

This shows that, prior to cross-clamping, the patient's acid-base status was normal – both the pH and the $PaCO_2$ were within the normal range.

Another arterial blood gas sample was sent off 30 minutes after the aorta was clamped and the results were: a pH of 7.13, pCO_2 of 6.66kPa (49.9mmHg), pO_2 of 6.3kPa (.6mmHg), HCO_3 of 23, and BE of 2.2

Six-step ABG interpretation of case study 5.1

Step 1: Review the patient   Given the information in the above scenario, hypoperfusion has resulted in increasing hypoxia of the tissues.
Step 2: Analyse the oxygenation   The O_2 and SaO_2 are low. Oxygen increased.
Step 3: Assess the pH   The pH indicates acidemia.
Step 4: Assess for respiratory disturbance   The pCO_2 is normal high.
Step 5: Assess for metabolic disturbance   The HCO_3 and BE are low and go in the opposite direction to the pH; the primary problem is therefore metabolic.

Step 6: Establish if the disturbance is compensatory or mixed
N/A
Interpretation:
Metabolic acidosis.

The patient now has hypoperfusion, due to a cessation in blood flow via the major vessels distal to the aortic clamp. This results in increasing hypoxia of the tissues, along with simultaneous hyperperfusion proximal to the cross-clamping. There is a shift in the distribution of the circulation blood volume and an increased load upon the cardiac system during this time. The ABG results show a developing metabolic acidosis as the distal tissues receive less oxygen. Aortic clamping at the infra-renal level is associated with a decrease in renal blood flow, decreasing blood flow though the kidneys by up to 30% (Gelman 1995).

In this case study, the signs and symptoms generally associated with metabolic acidosis are not visible as they are masked by the anaesthetic. In other examples, the symptoms would manifest as gastrointestinal effects of nausea and vomiting and abdominal pain. The nervous system effects would include weakness, lethargy, confusion, stupor, coma and depression of vital functions. The cardiovascular effects that may be seen in an awake patient are peripheral vasodilatation, bradycardia or a slower than normal heart rate and cardiac arrhythmias. All these symptoms may be presented by patients for a number of conditions and definitive diagnosis must therefore only be made after a thorough assessment. Signs that a patient may be compensating are: an increase in respiratory rate and depth, hyperkalemia, acid in the urine and increased ammonia in the urine. Investigations that will indicate a metabolic acidosis in all patients will be arterial blood gas results to identify a decrease in blood pH, bicarbonate (HCO_3 – an early sign) and PCO_2 (a sign of compensation) (Porth 2010).

The reduction in distal tissue perfusion and increasing hypoxia result in an increasing lactic acidosis due to anaerobic cellular perfusion. The normal method of lactic acid removal will be via the kidneys, through the angiotensin cycle. In this scenario, the normal buffering system to maintain homeostasis is insufficient and a metabolic acidosis develops. The normal range for blood pH that is compatible with life is 7.35 to 7.45. This patient has a decreasing pH and an increasing acidosis. The consequences of such a situation can include dysrhythmias and impaired cardiac conduction. A pH of 6.8 is usually incompatible with life (Clarke & Ketchell 2011).

Once the aneurysm has been repaired, the aortic clamps will be removed. This will be a critical time for the patient – after a prolonged tissue hypoxia reperfusion flushes out lactate from the cells.

Upon release of the aortic clamps, the anaesthetist requests another arterial blood gas test and this shows a much greater metabolic disorder than before.

A normal physiological response would be to address this metabolic acidosis with both renal and respiratory effort. The kidneys would excrete bicarbonate and the patient would hyperventilate to excrete CO_2. However, as the patient is ventilated, the end tidal CO_2 would display a sharp rise in pulmonary CO_2 levels as the patient's circulatory system restores perfusion to the tissues distal to the aortic repair.

The priority here is to monitor the patient closely, as this situation is a transient metabolic acidosis resulting from an ischemic episode due to the reduced blood flow. Attempts to hasten the correction with rapid reperfusion may make the situation worse. However, there is a 5.4% risk of renal impairment (Kumar 2002) following this type of surgery, and patients should be monitored closely for signs and symptoms of renal deficit.

This case study has looked at the development of metabolic acidosis as a result of lactic acid accumulation due to hypoxia during a surgical intervention. In other acute care settings, a similar lactic acidosis scenario may develop as a result of septic or cardiogenic shock (Kumar 2002).

Case study 5.2

A 24-year-old male motorist is brought to the emergency department by ambulance following a high-speed collision with a tree. The patient has intravenous 0.9% saline fluids in place following cannulation by the paramedic on scene. The patient presents with a pulse of 120, blood pressure of 110/65, a respiratory rate of 24 and a temperature of 35°C. The patient is alert and communicating with staff.

Case study 5.2: Assessment and treatment

On initial examination, the patient has a suspected right distal tibial fracture, and severe bruising over the abdomen and the right clavicle consistent with seatbelt use. During the initial examination, airway is fine, with no injuries. Breathing is rapid and shallow and rate is increasing to 26 rpm. The circulation is assessed and pulse rate is 130, with BP of 132/60. Capillary refill is >3s and the patient's temperature is 35°C. Haemoglobin (Hb) is measured by HemoCue as being 11.

The patient is taken to the operating theatre following an abdominal assessment showing free blood in the abdominal cavity. An emergency laparotomy reveals that the patient has extensive blood loss due to a mesenteric bleed. An ABG is taken and shows a pH of 6.95, pCO_2 of 5.55 kPa (41.6mmHg), pO_2 of 41.4 kPa (310.5mmHg), HCO_3 of 8.9mmol/l and BE of 1.

Six-step ABG interpretation of case study 5.2

Step 1: Review the patient
Given the information in the above scenario, there is severe tissue hypoxia due to hypovolemia.
Step 2: Analyse the oxygenation
The O_2 and SaO_2 are low, and oxygen is supplemented.
Step 3: Assess the pH
The pH indicates acidemia.

Step 4: Assess for respiratory disturbance
The pCO$_2$ is normal high.

Step 5: Assess for metabolic disturbance
The HCO$_3$ and BE are low and go in the same direction as the pH; the primary problem is therefore metabolic.

Step 6: Establish if the disturbance is compensatory or mixed.
N/A

Interpretation:
Metabolic acidosis.

The patient is in a severe metabolic acidosis, with decreasing Hb due to hypovolemia. This in turn creates severe tissue hypoxia.

References

Clarke, D. & Ketchell, A. (2011). *Nursing the Acutely Ill Adult: Priorities in assessment and management*. Basingstoke: Palgrave Macmillan.

Gelman, S. (1995). The pathophysiology of aortic cross-clamping and unclamping. *Anaesthesiology*. **82**, 1026–57.

Kumar, P.C.M. (2002). *Clinical Medicine*. 5th edn. Edinburgh: W.B. Saunders.

Porth, C.M.M.G. (2010). *Essesntials of Pathophysiology: concepts of altered health states*. 3rd revised North American Edition edn. Philadelphia: Lippincott Williams and Wilkins.

Tobias, J.R.P.R.J. (October 2006). An evaluation of acid base changes following aortic cross-clamping using transcutaneous carbon dioxide monitoring. *Pediatric Cardiology*. **27**, 585–88.

6

Metabolic alkalosis
Stanley Swanepoel

Causes of metabolic alkalosis

Metabolic alkalosis has been shown to contribute to 50% of hospitalised acid-base disorders (Kumar 2002). These findings are consistent with the prevalence of vomiting, suction and the use of diuretics within the clinical hospital setting. There is an associated mortality rate of 45% in patients with an arterial pH of 7.55; and this rises to 80% when the pH is above 7.65. When a severe metabolic alkalosis presents, it should be viewed with concern and treatment should be based upon the underlying causes. Some of these causes are shown in Table 6.1 (below).

Table 6.1 Common causes of metabolic alkalosis

Chloride depletion:
- Gastric losses (vomiting, mechanical drainage, bulimia)
- Chloruretic diuretics (bumetanide, chlorothiazide, metolazone, etc.)
- Diarrheal states (villous adenoma, congenital chloridorrhea)
- Posthypercapneic state
- Dietary chloride deprivation with base loading (chloride-deficient infant formulas)
- Gastrocystoplasty
- Cystic fibrosis (high sweat chloride).

Potassium depletion/mineralocorticoid excess:
- Primary aldosteronism (adenoma, idiopathic, hyperplasia, renin-responsive, glucocorticoid-suppressible, carcinoma)
- Apparent mineralocorticoid excess
  - Primary deoxycorticosterone excess (11β- and 17α-hydroxylase deficiencies)
  - Drugs: licorice (glycyrrhizic acid) as a confection or flavouring, carbenoxolone
  - Liddle syndrome

- Secondary aldosteronism
  - Adrenal corticosteroid excess (primary, secondary, exogenous)
  - Severe hypertension (malignant, accelerated, renovascular)
  - Hemangiopericytoma, nephroblastoma, renal cell carcinoma
- Bartter and Gitelman syndromes and their variants
- Laxative abuse, clay ingestion.

Hypercalcemic states:
- Hypercalcemia of malignancy
- Acute or chronic milk-alkali syndrome

Other:
- Carbenicillin, ampicillin, penicillin
- Bicarbonate ingestion (massive or with renal insufficiency)
- Recovery from starvation
- Hypoalbuminemia

Case study 6.1

In this scenario we will look at metabolic alkalosis. Consider a 74-year-old woman who has been admitted to hospital following a fall at home. The patient is frail and lives alone and was not found for 6 hours following her fall. On examination, she is found to be dehydrated and normothermic (37.2°C) although a mild urinary tract infection is present. She has severe bruising to her right hip but has not sustained any fractures.

Central nervous system signs of a metabolic alkalosis are: hyperactive reflexes, tetany, confusion and seizures. However, in an elderly patient, the presentation of confusion may not initially indicate a metabolic disorder, as there could be other possible factors to consider. The cardiovascular effects of hypotension and cardiac arrhythmias may also be masked by pre-existing conditions. Signs of compensation for a metabolic alkalosis are a decrease in respiratory rate and depth, leading to varying degrees of hypoxia and a resultant respiratory acidosis as the body conserves CO_2 (Porth 2010).

Case study 6.1: Assessment and treatment

The patient is placed on a care of the elderly ward and is on an intravenous and oral fluid regime to begin correcting her dehydration.

After 24 hours in hospital, the patient develops diarrhoea and vomiting. This continues for 6 hours and the medical staff request an arterial blood gas sample to be taken as part of her systematic assessment. The results show a pH of 7.45, pCO_2 of 5.5kPa (41.2mmHg), pO_2 of 14.6kPa (109.5mmHg), HCO_3 of 20 and BE of 4.

The diarrhoea and vomiting continue for another 6 hours and the patient becomes increasingly dehydrated and there is a decrease in her sensorium. A repeat ABG measurement shows a pH of 7.43, pCO_2 of 5.5kPa (41.2mmHg), pO_2 of 12.5kPa (93.7mmHg), HCO_3 of 27 and BE of 7.

Six-step ABG interpretation of case study 6.1

Step 1: Review the patient Given the information in the above scenario, what is known is that vomiting will deplete the acids present in the stomach.
Step 2: Analyse the oxygenation The O_2 and SaO_2 are within range.
Step 3: Assess the pH The pH indicates alkalemia.
Step 4: Assess for respiratory disturbance The pCO_2 is normal.
Step 5: Assess for metabolic disturbance The HCO_3 and BE are high and go in the same direction as the pH; the primary problem is therefore metabolic.
Step 6: Establish if the disturbance is compensatory or mixed N/A
Interpretation: Metabolic alkalosis.

The effects of this situation are that the vomiting will deplete the acids present in the stomach (HCL, Na and K^+). Bicarbonate is generated as the body replaces these lost gastric fluids acids, thus adding to the plasma bicarbonate levels. The net level of HCO_3^- throughout the body will rise. The pH will often be close to or above 7.45 and the HCO_3^- will rise to above 28mEq/l. In order to rectify the increases in bicarbonate levels, the kidney will excrete more HCO_3^- and the need to conserve CO_2, in order to raise the PCO_2, will result in a reduced respiratory rate.

This shows that the patient is now in a state of metabolic alkalosis with a reduced respiratory rate, increased confusion, elevated pH and HCO_3^-, and a reduced SaO_2 and PCO_2.

Case study 6.2

A thin, frail 65-year-old woman was admitted to hospital with at least a 10-day history of abdominal pain and vomiting. She was mildly confused and unable to confirm the duration of her illness. She lived alone, was self-caring and was on no medication. Her general health was good and there was no history of cardiac, renal or chest disease.

Case study 6.2: Assessment and treatment

On admission to the emergency department, her assessment showed that there was free gas under the diaphragm, visible on an x-ray. Her ECG showed sinus rhythm and the amylase level was low. Surgical assessment of the patient was a presentation of bowel perforation with dehydration. The initial blood results in the emergency department showed a pH of 7.43, pO_2 of 12.5kPa (93.7mmHg), pCO_2 of 5.5kPa (41.2mmHg), HCO_3 of 27 and BE of 7.

Six-step ABG interpretation of case study 6.2

Step 1: Review the patient Given the information in the above scenario, the patient has bowel perforation and vomiting and is showing signs of dehydration.
Step 2: Analyse the oxygenation The O_2 and SaO_2 are within range.
Step 3: Assess the pH The pH indicates alkalemia.
Step 4: Assess for respiratory disturbance The pCO_2 is normal.
Step 5: Assess for metabolic disturbance The HCO_3 and BE are high and go in the same direction as the pH; the primary problem is therefore metabolic.
Step 6: Establish if the disturbance is compensatory or mixed N/A
Interpretation: Metabolic alkalosis.

This early arterial blood gas sample shows a metabolic alkalosis.

The patient is transferred to the operating theatre the same day for an emergency laparotomy where an abscess secondary to a ruptured appendix is discovered and resected.

During the perioperative phase, another arterial blood gas sample is taken and the results show a pH of 7.32, pO_2 of 10.7kPa (80.2mmHg), pCO_2 of 5.9kPa (44.2mmHg), HCO_3 of 22 and BE of 6.

The pH is dropping and the HCO_3 is dropping as the fluid resuscitation, with potassium, has begun to help restore normal intravascular volume.

References

Clarke, D. & Ketchell, A. (2011). *Nursing the Acutely Ill Adult: Priorities in assessment and management*. Basingstoke: Palgrave Macmillan.

Gelman, S. (1995). The pathophysiology of aortic cross-clamping and unclamping. *Anaesthesiology*. **82**, 1026–57.

Kumar, P.C.M. (2002). *Clinical Medicine*. 5th edn. Edinburgh: W.B. Saunders.

Porth, C.M.M.G. (2010). *Essesntials of Pathophysiology: concepts of altered health states*. 3rd revised North American Edition edn. Philadelphia: Lippincott Williams and Wilkins.

Tobias, J.R.P.R.J. (October 2006). An evaluation of acid base changes following aortic cross-clamping using transcutaneous carbon dioxide monitoring. *Pediatric Cardiology*. **27**, 585–88.

7

Compensatory mechanisms
Donna Pierre

When a respiratory or metabolic acid-base disturbance exists over a period of time, the body will attempt to counteract this through compensation. Compensation is achieved using the organ that is not the primary cause of the disturbance and depending on the functioning of the lungs, the kidneys and the severity of the disturbance. For example, if the disturbance is respiratory, the kidneys will compensate by either holding on to or releasing bicarbonate. Alternatively, if the disturbance is metabolic, the lungs will compensate by either blowing off or retaining CO_2. The aim of compensation is to return the pH to its normal range. However, neither the respiratory system nor the metabolic system has the ability to over-compensate (cause the pH to go above its normal range).

Acid-base disturbances can be uncompensated, partially compensated, or fully compensated. The case studies used in previous chapters are examples of uncompensated disturbances, where the pH showed acidosis or alkalosis, the disturbance was easily identified and the values for the compensatory system remained within range. In partially compensated gases, the pH and both the metabolic and respiratory markers are out of range, as the body makes a clear attempt to compensate, using the opposing organ. A quick guide to partially compensated ABGs is provided in Table 7.1 (below). Eventually, if the compensatory response causes the pH to return to normal range (though this is rare), the disturbance is described as 'fully compensated'. However, the other values may be abnormal.

Table 7.1 Causes and compensatory effects of acid-base disturbances

Disturbance	pH	Primary cause	Compensatory effect
Respiratory acidosis	Low	CO_2 high	HCO_3 high
Respiratory alkalosis	High	CO_2 low	HCO_3 low
Metabolic acidosis	Low	HCO_3 low	pCO_2 low
Metabolic alkalosis	High	HCO_3 high	pCO_2 high

Case study 7.1

Post abdominal surgery, Patient A arrives at the recovery unit with a fentanyl and bupivacaine epidural in situ. The block, when measured, is between T5 and L2, with a respiratory rate of 6 breaths per minute (bpm), saturation of 96% on 5l of oxygen via the non-rebreathe mask, with a blood pressure of 95/50mmHg and a heart rate of 67 beats per minute.

A routine ABG result shows a pH of 7.32, PO_2 of 11.0kPa (82.5mmHg), SaO_2 of 95%, PCO_2 of 6.9kPa (51.7mmHg), HCO_3^- of 34 and BE of -7.

Six-step ABG interpretation of case study 7.1

Step 1: Review the patient Given the information in the above scenario, the level of the block can lead to inefficiencies in respiratory muscles (Sasaki 2013), which would account for the low respiratory rate. A low respiratory rate (hypoventilation) will lead to the accumulation of CO_2.
Step 2: Analyse the oxygenation The O_2 and SaO_2 are within normal range.
Step 3: Assess the pH The pH indicates acidemia.
Step 4: Assess for respiratory disturbance The pCO_2 is elevated; the primary problem is therefore with the respiratory system.
Step 5: Assess for metabolic disturbance The HCO_3 and BE are elevated, but go in the opposite direction to the pH and therefore indicate that the metabolic system is compensating.
Step 6: Establish if the disturbance is compensatory or mixed Partially compensated, as the pH has not returned to normal.
Interpretation: Partially compensated respiratory acidosis.

Case study 7.2

An 80kg patient is admitted onto the ward for incision and drainage of a groin abscess. Whilst having 80ml per hour of Hartmann's infusing intravenously, clinical observations indicate 10ml of urine for the last 3 hours, blood pressure at 75/45, HR 138 and saturating at 92% on room air. Whilst urgent care intervention proceeds, an ABG reveals a pH of 7.31, $PaCO_2$ of 4.0kPa (30mmHg), PaO_2 of 9.6kPa (72mmHg), SaO_2 of 91, BE of −13 and HCO_3 of 17.

Six-step ABG interpretation of case study 7.2

Step 1: Review the patient Given the information in the above scenario, there is a degree of hypoperfusion, leading to low urine out (Legrand & Paven 2011).

Step 2: Analyse the oxygenation The O_2 and SaO_2 are low so oxygen therapy is commenced, as the patient has no history of respiratory disease.
Step 3: Assess the pH The pH indicates acidemia.
Step 4: Assess for respiratory disturbance The pCO_2 is low, but as this goes in the same direction as the pH, the respiratory system is compensating.
Step 5: Assess for metabolic disturbance The H_2O and BE are low, and go in the same direction as the pH; the primary problem is therefore metabolic.
Step 6: Establish if the disturbance is compensatory or mixed Partially compensated as the pH has not returned to normal.
Interpretation: Partially compensated metabolic acidosis.

Case study 7.3

Patient B arrives at the emergency department complaining of chest pain. Whilst the treatment for acute coronary syndrome is being implemented, the patient complains of feeling very nervous and anxious. Her heart rate is 140 bpm, blood pressure is 140/85, respiratory rate R 44 with saturations of 99% on 1l oxygen. A routine ABG reveals a pH of 7.49, $PaCO_2$ of 3.6kPa (27mmHg), PaO_2 of 13kPa (97.5mmHg), SaO_2 of 99.6%, BE of -5 and HCO_3 of 18.

Six-step ABG interpretation of case study 7.3

Step 1: Review the patient Given the information in the above scenario, the patient's anxiety caused hyperventilation, which is noted as an increase in respiratory rate. This then leads to an increase in the amount of CO_2 exhaled (Folgering 1999).
Step 2: Analyse the oxygenation The O_2 and SaO_2 are normal.
Step 3: Assess the pH The pH indicates alkalemia.
Step 4: Assess for respiratory disturbance The pCO_2 is low, and goes in the same direction as the pH; the respiratory system is therefore the primary problem.
Step 5: Assess for metabolic disturbance The HCO_3 and BE are also low, which indicates that the metabolic system is compensating.
Step 6: Establish if the disturbance is compensatory or mixed Partially compensated, as the pH has not returned to normal.

> **Interpretation:**
> Partially compensated respiratory alkalosis.

Case study 7.4

Patient C is admitted onto the medical assessment unit by his case worker, who reports that the patient has taken an overdose of Gaviscon. He is normally fit and well, with complaints of intermittent heartburn and a background history of schizophrenia.

His clinical observations are within his normal range. However, a routine ABG shows a pH of 7.48, $PaCO_2$ of 6.6kPa (49.5mmHg), PaO_2 of 13kPa (97.5mmHg), BE of +8 and HCO_3 of 38.

Six-step ABG interpretation of case study 7.4

Step 1: Review the patient
Given the information in the above scenario, excessive intake of bicarbonate (such as antacids) can cause alkalosis (Lewis 2016).

Step 2: Analyse the oxygenation
The O_2 and SaO_2 are normal.

Step 3: Assess the pH
The pH indicates alkalemia.

Step 4: Assess for respiratory disturbance
The pCO_2 is high, but it goes in the same direction as the pH; the respiratory system is therefore compensating.

Step 5: Assess for metabolic disturbance
The HCO_3 and BE are high, and go in the same direction as the pH; the primary problem is therefore metabolic.

Step 6: Establish if the disturbance is compensatory or mixed
Partially compensated, as the pH has not returned to normal.

Interpretation:
Partially compensated metabolic alkalosis.

Mixed acid-base disturbances

Mixed disturbances can occur if there is more than one primary acid-base disturbance present, such that both the $PaCO_2$ and HCO_3 are adding to the change in pH. In order to diagnose a mixed acid-base disorder, clinicians must have a thorough knowledge of the primary disturbance and the compensatory response.

Case study 7.5

Patient D was reported missing. After three days, she was found unconscious and collapsed, having sustained a fall. She was intubated and ventilated by the paramedics. On arrival at the hospital, she is taken to the operating theatre for examination under anaesthesia of an ischemic foot related to a broken ankle.

Prior to surgery, ABG results showed a pH of 6.9, PCO_2 of 13.2kPa (99mmHg), PO_2 of 15kPa (112.5mmHg) (on 100% oxygen), SaO_2 of 99%, HCO_3 of 14 and BE of -7.

Six-step ABG interpretation of case study 7.5

Step 1: Review the patient Given the information in the above scenario, the cause of the acidosis could be respiratory from hypoventilation or metabolic due to lactic acidosis from the ischemic limb (Andersen *et al.* 2013).
Step 2: Analyse the oxygenation The O_2 and SaO_2 are normal.
Step 3: Assess the pH The pH indicates acidemia.
Step 4: Assess for respiratory disturbance The pCO_2 is high, and goes in the opposite direction to the pH; the respiratory system is therefore the primary disorder.
Step 5: Assess for metabolic disturbance The HCO_3 and BE are low, and go in the opposite direction to the pH; the primary problem is therefore metabolic.
Step 6: Establish if the disturbance is compensatory or mixed Mixed disturbance.
Interpretation: Combined acidosis.

Case study 7.6

Patient E was admitted into hospital due to an exacerbation of chronic obstructive pulmonary disease (COPD) and was commenced on antibiotics. A chest x-ray showed diffuse pulmonary oedema and a furosemide infusion was commenced. Within the last 2 hours, the patient has passed >2l of urine and is now hypotensive. The outreach team is called. On investigation, a routine ABG shows a pH of 7.36, $PaCO_2$ of 7.4kPa (55.5mmHg), PaO_2 of 10kPa (75mmHg) on 4l of oxygen, SaO_2 of 94%, HCO_3 of 33 and BE of -6.

Six-step ABG interpretation of case study 7.6

Step 1: Review the patient Given the information in the above scenario, a known history of COPD indicates a higher CO_2 level. As furosemide is a non-potassium-sparing diuretic, hypokalemia could be expected as a consequence of the large urine output (Klabunde 2012).

Step 2: Analyse the oxygenation The O_2 and SaO_2 are normal for a patient with COPD.	
Step 3: Assess the pH The pH is normal (this can either indicate a normal, a compensated or mixed disturbance).	
Step 4: Assess for respiratory disturbance The pCO_2 is high but the pH is normal.	
Step 5: Assess for metabolic disturbance The HCO_3 and BE are high, but the pH is normal.	
Step 6: Establish if the disturbance is compensatory or mixed Mixed disturbance.	
Interpretation: Mixed respiratory acidosis and metabolic alkalosis.	

Case study 7.7

A patient with known cirrhosis of the liver has been admitted onto the liver unit due to increased shortness of breath, increased abdominal girth and severe swelling in all limbs. An abdominal x-ray confirms ascites. Whilst waiting for a drain insertion, intravenous diuretics have been administered. An admission ABG shows a pH of 7.48, PCO_2 of 3.8kPa (28.5mmHg), PaO_2 of 11kPa (82.5mmHg), SaO_2 of 96% on 28% oxygen, HCO_3 of 36 and BE of -9.

Six-step ABG interpretation of case study 7.7

Step 1: Review the patient Given the information in the above scenario, metabolic alkalosis is often found in patients with liver disease on diuretic therapy (Rabelink 1999), or patients with increased urinary H^+ loss, or those with a degree of hyperventilation.
Step 2: Analyse the oxygenation The O_2 and SaO_2 are within range.
Step 3: Assess the pH The pH indicates alkalosis.
Step 4: Assess for respiratory disturbance The pCO_2 is low and goes in the opposite direction to the pH; the respiratory system is therefore the primary disorder.
Step 5: Assess for metabolic disturbance The HCO_3 and BE are high and go in the same direction as the pH; the metabolic system is therefore the primary disorder.
Step 6: Establish if the disturbance is compensatory or mixed Mixed disturbance.

Interpretation: Combined alkalosis.

Case study 7.8

Patient G has been admitted to hospital complaining of chest tightness and a productive cough on a background of chronic renal failure. A chest x-ray has confirmed pneumonia. Whilst his current clinical observations remain stable, his respiratory rate is 38bpm and a routine ABG shows a pH of 7.39, pCO_2 of 3.9kPa (29.2mmHg), PO_2 of 10.0kPa (75mmHg), SaO_2 of 96%, HCO_3 of 18 and BE of -6.

Six-step ABG interpretation of case study 7.8

Step 1: Review the patient Given the information in the above scenario, the chronic renal failure may cause an acidosis, due to the inability of the kidneys to regulate bicarbonate (Kovesdy 2012). The noted hyperventilation may also cause an increase in the amount of CO_2 exhaled.
Step 2: Analyse the oxygenation The O_2 and SaO_2 are within range.
Step 3: Assess the pH The pH is normal (this can indicate a normal, compensated or mixed disturbance).
Step 4: Assess for respiratory disturbance The pCO_2 is low, confirming a respiratory alkalosis.
Step 5: Assess for metabolic disturbance The HCO_3 and BE are low, confirming an increase in metabolic acids.
Step 6: Establish if the disturbance is compensatory or mixed Mixed disturbance.
Interpretation: Respiratory alkalosis with metabolic acidosis.

References

Andersen, L.W., Mackenhauer, J., Roberts, J.C., Berg, K.M., Cocchi, M.N. & Donnino, M.W. (2013). Etiology and therapeutic approach to elevated lactate. *Mayo Clinic Proceedings.* **88**(10), 1127–40.

Folgering, H. (1999). The pathophysiology of hyperventilation syndrome. *Monaldi Archives for Chest Disease.* **54**(4), 365–72.

Klabunde, R.E. (2012). *Cardiovascular Pharmacology Concepts*
http://www.cvpharmacology.com/diuretic/diuretics (accessed 30 June 2016).

Kovesdy, C.P. (2012). Metabolic acidosis and kidney disease: does bicarbonate therapy slow the progression of CKD? *Nephrology Dialysis Transplantation.* **27**(8), 3056–62.

Legrand, M. & Payen, D. (2011). Understanding urine output in critically ill patients. *Annals of Intensive Care.* **1**(13), 1–8.

Lewis, J.L. (2016). *Metabolic Alkalosis.* http://www.merckmanuals.com/professional/endocrine-and-metabolic-disorders/acid-base-regulation-and-disorders/metabolic-alkalosis (accessed 30 June 2016).

Rabelink, T.J. (1999). Acid-base abnormalities in a patient with hepatic chirrhosis. *Nephrology Dialysis Transplantation.* **14**, 1599–1601.

Sasaki, N., Meyer, M.J. & Eikermann, M. (2013). Postoperative Respiratory Muscle Dysfunction: Pathophysiology and preventative strategies. *Anaesthesiology.* **118**(4), 961–78.

8

ABG analysis practice questions and answers

Reference ranges

pH   7.35–7.45
PaO$_2$ 11.5–13.5kPa (86.2–101.2mmHg)
PaCO$_2$ 4.5–6.0kPa (33.7–45mmHg)
HCO$_3$ 22–28 mmol/l
BE   -2 to +2
SaO$_2$ 98%

Case study 8.1

A 17-year-old semi-comatose diabetic patient arrives in A & E with Kussmaul breathing. His ABG on room air is shown below. How would you interpret the results?

pH   7.05
PaO$_2$ 14.4kPa (108mmHg)
PaCO$_2$ 1.6kPa (12mmHg)
HCO$_3$ 5mmol/l
BE   -10
SaO$_2$ 98%

Case study 8.2

A 20-year-old male is admitted to hospital after taking an overdose of barbiturates. His ABG on room air is shown below. How would you interpret the results?

pH   7.18
PaO$_2$ 8.0kPa (60mmHg)
PaCO$_2$ 8.0kPa (60mmHg)

HCO₃   25mmol/l

BE   0

SaO₂   74%

Case study 8.3

An 18-year-old girl arrives in A & E complaining of malaise and vomiting over the last few days. She says she feels tingly and shaky. Her ABG on room air is shown below. How would you interpret the result?

pH   7.55

PaO₂   11.3kPa (84.7mmHg)

PaCO₂   8.7kPa (65.2mmHg)

HCO₃   31mmol/l

BE   +7

SaO₂   98%

Case study 8.4

A 35-year-old male patient with pneumonia is being ventilated on ITU. He has a respiratory rate of 12 and is receiving 80% oxygen. His latest ABG is shown below. How would you interpret the result?

pH   7.36

PaO₂   11.46kPa (85.9mmHg)

PaCO₂   8.7kPa (65.2mmHg)

HCO₃   37mmol/l

BE   +10

SaO₂   96%

Case study 8.5

A 62-year-old man is receiving 4 litres of oxygen on the ward after a liver resection. He developed renal failure postoperatively and received haemofiltration for two days. His latest ABG is shown below. How would you interpret the result?

pH   7.49

PaO₂   12.3kPa (92.2mmHg)

PaCO₂   5.2kPa (39mmHg)

HCO₃   31mmol/l

BE   +6

SaO₂   98%

Case study 8.6

A 57-year-old man with hypovolemic shock, following ruptured oesophageal varices, has had a cardiac arrest on the ward. His ABG immediately after resuscitation is shown below. How would you interpret the result?

pH	6.9
PaO_2	12.4kPa (93mmHg)
$PaCO_2$	13.7kPa (102.7mmHg)
HCO_3	19mmol/l
BE	-10
SaO_2	97%

Case study 8.7

A 63-year-old man with liver cirrhosis and ascites is being treated with diuretics. An ABG reveals the results below. How would you interpret his ABG?

pH	7.6
PaO_2	13.0kPa (97.5mmHg)
$PaCO_2$	3.0kPa (22.5mmHg)
HCO_3	33mmol/l
BE	+8
SaO_2	96%

Case study 8.8

A 76-year-old woman is admitted to the orthopaedic ward, following a fall that resulted in a fractured neck of femur. She has a fruity odour to her breath. Her ABG result is shown below. How would you interpret the result?

pH	7.32
PaO_2	11.1kPa (83.2mmHg)
$PaCO_2$	4.0kPa (30mmHg)
HCO_3	18mmol/l
BE	-6
SaO_2	95%

Case study 8.9

A 28-year-old man is admitted for a routine inguinal hernia repair. Prior to surgery, he is anxious and has a respiratory rate of 42bpm. He complains that his fingers are tingling. How would you interpret the ABG results below?

pH	7.50
PaO_2	13.3kPa (99.7mmHg)
$PaCO_2$	3.7kPa (27.7mmHg)
HCO_3	25mmol/l
BE	+1
SaO_2	95%

Case study 8.10

A 27-year-old man is admitted to the HDU via A & E following a road traffic accident. He has two compound fractures of the left leg and multiple rib fractures. Shortly after admission, he complains of severe pain on inspiration. His respirations are shallow, with a rate of 38bpm. His ABG is presented below. How would you interpret the results?

pH	7.33
PaO_2	9.9kPa (74.2mmHg)
$PaCO_2$	7.3kPa (54.7mmHg)
HCO_3	28mmol/l
BE	+4
SaO_2	92%

Arterial blood gas (ABG) analysis practice (answers)

Six-step ABG interpretation of case study 8.1

Step 1: Review the patient
From the history, it could be noted that the patient is diabetic, with reduced conscious level, and his breathing is laboured. However, reduced conscious levels should cause a decrease in respiratory rate.
Step 2: Analyse the oxygenation
The PaO_2 and SaO_2 are within normal range.
Step 3: Assess the pH
The pH is indicative of acidosis.
Step 4: Assess for respiratory disturbance
The $PaCO_2$ is low due to the increase in respiratory rate. However, a low CO_2 causes an increase in pH; the primary problem is not therefore respiratory.
Step 5: Assess for metabolic disturbance
The HCO_3 and BE are also low, and go in the same direction as the pH; the primary problem is therefore metabolic.

Step 6: Establish if the disturbance is compensatory or mixed
Partially compensated by the respiratory system due to the low PCO_2 and the pH has not returned to normal range.

Interpretation:
Partially compensated metabolic acidosis.

Six-step ABG interpretation of case study 8.2

Step 1: Review the patient
From the history, the patient has taken an overdose of barbiturates, which are a sedative-hypnotic class of medication. An overdose can cause respiratory depression.

Step 2: Analyse the oxygenation
The PaO_2 and SaO_2 are low (administer oxygen).

Step 3: Assess the pH
The pH is low and is indicative of acidosis.

Step 4: Assess for respiratory disturbance
The $PaCO_2$ is high, possibly due to the decrease in respiratory rate, causing a raise in CO_2 levels. A high CO_2 causes a decrease in pH; the primary problem is therefore respiratory.

Step 5: Assess for metabolic fisturbance
The HCO_3 and BE are within normal range.

Step 6: Establish if the disturbance is compensatory or mixed
N/A

Interpretation:
Respiratory acidosis.

Six-step ABG interpretation of case study 8.3

Step 1: Review the patient
From the history, the patient has complained of vomiting, which causes a loss of acids.

Step 2: Analyse the oxygenation
The PaO_2 is within range.

Step 3: Assess the pH
The pH is high and is indicative of alkalosis.

Step 4: Assess for respiratory disturbance
The $PaCO_2$ is high. However, a high CO_2 causes a decrease in pH; the primary problem is therefore not respiratory.

Step 5: Assess for metabolic disturbance
The HCO_3 and BE are high, and go in the same direction as the pH; the primary problem is therefore metabolic.

Step 6: Establish if the disturbance is compensatory or mixed
Partially compensated by the respiratory system due to the high PCO_2, and the pH is not within range.

Interpretation:
Partially compensated metabolic alkalosis.

Six-step ABG interpretation of case study 8.4

Step 1: Review the patient
From the history, the patient has pneumonia, which may impair his CO_2 and O_2 exchange.

Step 2: Analyse the oxygenation
The PaO_2 and SaO_2 are within range.

Step 3: Assess the pH
The pH is within range, and this can indicate a normal, compensated or mixed disturbance.

Step 4: Assess for respiratory disturbance
The $PaCO_2$ is high, and a high CO_2 causes a decrease in pH. The ideal pH is 7.4. However, in this case, the pH can be described as acidotic, although only just within range.

Step 5: Assess for metabolic disturbance
The HCO_3 and BE are high but go in the opposite direction to the pH; the primary problem is therefore not metabolic.

Step 6: Establish if the disturbance is compensatory or mixed
Compensated by the metabolic system, as the pH is within normal range.

Interpretation:
Compensated respiratory acidosis.

Six-step ABG interpretation of case study 8.5

Step 1: Review the patient
From the history, the patient is in renal failure, and the kidneys play an important role in acid-base balance.

Step 2: Analyse the oxygenation
The PaO_2 and SaO_2 are within range.

Step 3: Assess the pH
The pH is high and indicates alkalosis.

Step 4: Assess for respiratory disturbance
$PaCO_2$ is within range.

Step 5: Assess for metabolic disturbance
The HCO_3 and BE are high, and go in the same direction as the pH; the primary problem is therefore metabolic.

| Step 6: Establish if the disturbance is compensatory or mixed |
| N/A |

| Interpretation: |
| Metabolic alkalosis. |

Six-step ABG interpretation of case study 8.6

| **Step 1: Review the patient** |
| From the history, the patient is hypovolemic, which, at a cellular level, can lead to anaerobic metabolism, and the production of lactate acid. A cardiac arrest can cause carbon dioxide (an acid) to be retained in the body. |

| **Step 2: Analyse the oxygenation** |
| The PaO_2 and SaO_2 are within range. |

| **Step 3: Assess the pH** |
| The pH is low and indicates acidosis |

| **Step 4: Assess for respiratory disturbance** |
| The $PaCO_2$ is high, which causes a low pH; the primary problem is therefore respiratory. |

| **Step 5: Assess for metabolic disturbance** |
| The HCO_3 and BE are low, and go in the same direction as the pH; the primary problem is therefore metabolic. |

| **Step 6: Establish if the disturbance is compensatory or mixed** |
| N/A |

| **Interpretation:** |
| Mixed respiratory and metabolic acidosis. |

Six-step ABG interpretation of case study 8.7

| **Step 1: Review the patient** |
| From the history, the patient has ascites, indicating problems with the body's fluid distribution and therefore ion and cations distribution, which is further enhanced by the use of diuretics. |

| **Step 2: Analyse the oxygenation** |
| The PaO_2 and SaO_2 are within range. |

| **Step 3: Assess the pH** |
| The pH is low and indicates alkalosis. |

| **Step 4: Assess for respiratory disturbance** |
| The $PaCO_2$ is low, and a low CO_2 causes an increase in pH; the primary problem is therefore respiratory. |

| **Step 5: Assess for metabolic disturbance** |
| The HCO_3 and BE are high, but go in the opposite direction to the pH. |

Step 6: Establish if the disturbance is compensatory or mixed
Partially compensated by the metabolic system due to decreased HCO_3 and BE, and the pH being out of range.

Interpretation:
Partially compensated respiratory alkalosis.

Six-step ABG interpretation of case study 8.8

Step 1: Review the patient
From the history, the presentation of a 'fruity odour' breath is a sign of ketoacidosis, which may occur in diabetics.

Step 2: Analyse the oxygenation
The PaO_2 and SaO_2 are within range

Step 3: Assess the pH
The pH is low and indicates acidosis.

Step 4: Assess for respiratory disturbance
The $PaCO_2$ is within range.

Step 5: Assess for metabolic disturbance
The HCO_3 and BE are low, and go in the same direction as the pH; the primary problem is therefore metabolic.

Step 6: Establish if the disturbance is compensatory or mixed
N/A

Interpretation:
Metabolic acidosis.

Six-step ABG interpretation of case study 8.9

Step 1: Review the patient
From the history and clinical assessment, a high respiratory rate is noted, along with some effects on the nervous system.

Step 2: Analyse the oxygenation
The PaO_2 and SaO_2 are within range.

Step 3: Assess the pH
The pH is high and indicates alkalosis.

Step 4: Assess for respiratory disturbance
The $PaCO_2$ is low, and a low CO_2 causes an increase in pH; the primary problem is therefore respiratory.

Step 5: Assess for metabolic disturbance
The HCO_3 and BE are within range.

Step 6: Establish if the disturbance is compensatory or mixed
N/A

Interpretation:
Respiratory alkalosis.

Six-step ABG interpretation of case study 8.10

Step 1: Review the patient
From the history and clinical assessment, injuries from the RTA have caused damage to the mechanisms involved with breathing, which can lead to gas exchange impairment.

Step 2: Analyse the oxygenation
The PaO_2 and SaO_2 are low (administer oxygen).

Step 3: Assess the pH
The pH is low and indicates acidosis.

Step 4: Assess for respiratory disturbance
The $PaCO_2$ is high, and a high CO_2 causes a decrease in pH; the primary problem is therefore respiratory.

Step 5: Assess for metabolic disturbance
The HCO_3 is elevated and goes in the opposite direction to the pH. However, the BE is currently within range.

Step 6: Establish if the disturbance is compensatory or mixed
Partially compensated by the metabolic system, due to the increase in HCO_3. The pH has not yet returned to normal. The BE is currently within range. However, this will eventually follow the direction of the HCO_3.

Interpretation:
Partially compensated respiratory acidosis.

References

Aiken, C.G.A. (2013). History and medical understanding and misunderstanding of acid-base balance. *Journal of Clinical and Diagnostic Research.* **7**(9), 2038–41.

Atherton, J.C. (2009). Acid-base balance: maintenance of plasma pH. *Anaesthesia and Intensive Care.* **10**(11), 557–61.

Ayers, P. & Dixon, C. (2012). Simple acid-base tutorial. *Journal of Parenteral and Enteral Nutrition.* **36**(1), 18–23.

Ayers, P., Dixon, C. & Mays, A. (2015). Acid-base disorders: Learning the basics. *Nutrition in Clinical Practice.* **30**(1), 14–20.

Day, J. & Pandit, J.J. (2010). Analysis of blood gases and acid-base balance. *Surgery.* **29**(3), 107–11.

Edwards, S.L. (2008). Pathophysiology of acid-base balance: The theory practice relationship. *Intensive and Critical Care Nursing.* **24**, 28–40.

Rogers, K.M.A. & McCutcheon, K. (2013). Understanding arterial blood gases. *The Journal of Perioperative Practice.* **23**(9), 191–97.

Glossary of terms

acid substance having a pH of less than 7

acute respiratory distress syndrome medical condition occurring in critically ill patients, characterised by widespread inflammation in the lungs

alkaline substance having a pH greater than 7 and being capable of neutralising an acid

alveolar ventilation the total volume of gas entering the lungs per minute

amino-acid organic compound serving as a building block for proteins

amylase enzyme that facilitates carbohydrate digestion

analgesia medication that acts to relieve pain

anion atom or molecule with more electrons than protons, giving it a net negative charge

anion gap calculated value that represents the concentration of the unmeasured anions in the plasma

anxiety hyperventilation syndrome several physical and emotional symptoms largely brought about by over-breathing

aortic aneurysm enlargement (dilation) of the aorta to greater than 1.5 times normal size

ascites accumulation of fluid in the peritoneal cavity

asthma long-term inflammatory disease in the lungs

barbiturate drug that depresses the central nervous system, producing a wide range of effects, from mild sedation to total anaesthesia

benzodiazepine tranquiliser used to treat both anxiety and sleeping problems

bicarbonate (HCO_3) most important buffer in blood to help prevent development of acidosis

bradypnoeic abnormally low breathing rate

buffer component of a solution that can neutralise either an acid or a base and thus maintain a constant pH

bupivacaine drug used to produce local anaesthesia

cannula thin tube inserted into a vein or body cavity to administer medications/fluids, drain off fluid or insert a surgical instrument

carbon dioxide (CO_2) colourless, odourless incombustible gas

carbon monoxide colourless, odourless gas, slightly less dense than air

cation atom or molecule with fewer electrons than protons, giving it a net positive charge

central venous catheter catheter placed into a large central vein for the purpose of monitoring fluid balance and/or the administration of drugs and fluids

cerebrovascular accident (CVA) sudden death of some brain cells due to lack of oxygen when blood flow to the brain is impaired by thrombosis or haemorrhage

chronic bronchitis long-term inflammation of the bronchi in the lungs

chronic obstructive pulmonary disease (COPD) obstructive lung disease characterised by long-term poor airflow

cirrhosis scarring of the liver caused by continuous, long-term liver damage

compound fracture open wound where a fractured bone penetrates the skin

deep vein thrombosis (DVT) formation of a thrombus within a deep vein

dehydrated experiencing a deficit of total body water

diaphragm dome-shaped muscular partition separating the thorax from the abdomen

distal situated away from the centre of the body or from the point of attachment

diuretic drug that promotes the production of urine

diverticulitis inflammation of the diverticulum, especially in the colon, causing pain and disturbance of bowel function

dyspnoea difficulty with the act of breathing

dysrhythmia abnormality in a physiological rhythm, especially in the brain or heart

emphysema long-term progressive disease of the lungs

encephalitis acute inflammation of the brain

enzyme protein molecule that helps other organic molecules to enter into chemical reactions with one another but is itself unaffected by these reactions

epidural injection or infusion of local anaesthetic agent into the epidural space around the spinal cord

equilibrium maintaining equal balance

fentanyl synthetic opiate drug that is a powerful painkiller and tranquiliser

fibroid benign tumour of muscular and fibrous tissue, typically developing in the wall of the uterus

flail chest life-threatening condition when a segment of the rib cage fractures under stress and becomes detached from the rest of the chest wall

furosemide loop diuretic promoting fluid excretion in the Loop of Henle of the nephron

Gaviscon drug used to relieve the symptoms of acid indigestion/reflux

Guillain-Barré Syndrome rapid-onset muscle weakness caused by the immune system damaging the peripheral nervous system

haemofiltration renal replacement therapy used in critical care areas, often when treating acute kidney injury

haemoglobin (Hb) protein molecule in red blood cells

Hartmann's crystalloid solution that is most closely isotonic with blood

homeostasis tendency towards a relatively stable equilibrium

hydration act or process of combining or treating with water

hydrogen chemical element denoted by the chemical symbol H

hydroxylation introduction of hydroxyl into a compound

hyperkalemia potassium level in the blood that is higher than the set reference range

hypertension abnormally high blood pressure

hypocapnia reduced level of carbon dioxide in the blood

hypovolemic shock condition when the fluid volume of the circulatory system is too depleted to allow adequate circulation to the tissues of the body

hysterectomy surgical procedure to remove all or part of the uterus

inguinal hernia protrusion of abdominal cavity contents through the inguinal canal

ischemic restriction in blood supply to the tissues, causing a shortage of oxygen and glucose needed for cellular metabolism

ketone inorganic compound containing a carbonyl group bonded to two hydrocarbon groups

kilopascal (kPa) 1000 Newtons of pressure per square metre

Kussmaul breathing deep and laboured breathing pattern often associated with severe metabolic acidosis

kyphoscoliosis s-shaped deformity of the spine characterised by abnormal curvature of the vertebral column in two planes (coronal and sagittal)

lactic acid acid produced through a fermentation process during metabolism

laparotomy surgical procedure involving a large incision through the abdominal wall to gain access to the abdominal cavity

malaise general feeling of discomfort, illness or unease whose exact cause is difficult to identify

menorrhagia abnormally heavy bleeding during menstruation

metabolic processes employed in order to generate energy

minute volume volume of gas inhaled or exhaled from the lungs over a period of 1 minute

morphine narcotic, analgesic drug, derived from opium and used medicinally to relieve pain

motor neurone disease progressive disease involving degeneration of the motor neurons and wasting of the muscles

muscular dystrophy hereditary condition marked by progressive weakening and wasting of the muscles

myasthenia gravis condition causing abnormal weakness of certain muscles

myocardial infarction irreversible necrosis of myocardium secondary to prolonged lack of oxygen supply

naloxone competitive opioid antagonist drug

narcotic drug that induces drowsiness, stupor or insensibility and relieves pain

normothermic normal state of temperature

obesity medical condition in which excess body fat has accumulated to the extent that it may have an adverse effect on health

obstructive sleep apnoea complete or partial obstruction of the upper airway during sleep, leading to periods of apnoea

oesophageal varices abnormally dilated submucosal veins in the oesophagus

oxygen (O_2) colourless, odourless reactive gas

partial pressure refers to quantity of a gas and describes how much of a gas is present

phosphate building block for important substances such as cell membranes and DNA

phospholipid class of lipids that are a major component of cell membranes

plasma protein any of the various dissolved proteins of blood plasma, including antibodies and blood-clotting proteins that act by holding fluid in blood vessels by osmosis

pneumonia severe and complicated variety of chest infection

pneumothorax abnormal collection of air or gas in the pleural space that causes an uncoupling of lung from the chest wall

positive pressure ventilation provision of respiratory gases under pressure by a mechanical ventilator

pulmonary embolism blockage in the pulmonary artery caused by a substance that has travelled from elsewhere in the body

pulmonary oedema fluid accumulation in the alveoli of the lungs

pyrexia raised body temperature

SaO_2 indirect measurement of the amount of oxygen bound to haemoglobin in blood

schizophrenia mental health disorder characterised by abnormal social behaviour and failure to understand what is real

seizure physical findings or change in behaviour that occur after an episode of abnormal electrical activity in the brain

supra-tentorial pain, fear, stress, related to an area of the brain located above the tentorium cerebelli

tachycardia abnormally high heart rate

tetany condition characterised by muscular spasms of the hands and feets, cramps, laryngeal spasms and overactive neurological reflexes

thoracoplasty surgical remodelling or reshaping of the thorax

tidal volume volume of gas inhaled or exhaled from the lungs with each breath

volatile liable to change rapidly and unpredictably, usually for the worse

Index